Illness Isn't Caused By A Drug Deficiency!

"Of all the things man knows, he knows least about himself—how his body works, how to stay healthy and prevent disease, how his mind works and how to use it as a productive, creative tool, and the spiritual aspects of himself. In the area of technology, man has come a long way through the course of evolution, but in understanding himself, he has barely made any progress at all."

—Vic Shayne, Ph.D.

Illness Isn't Caused By A Drug Deficiency!

—Healthy Choices & Whole Nutrition

Vic Shayne, Ph.D.

Writers Club Press

San Jose New York Lincoln Shanghai

Illness Isn't Caused By A Drug Deficiency!
—Healthy Choices & Whole Nutrition

Writers Club Press
an imprint of iUniverse.com, Inc.

For information address:
iUniverse.com, Inc.
5220 S 16th, Ste. 200
Lincoln, NE 68512
www.iuniverse.com

Cover Photograph by R. Jones: Bolivia,1996:
"Vegetables on Sale at Sucre Market"

This book is not intended as a replacement for sound medical or healthcare advice, nor is it a guide for the treatment or cure of disease. Always consult your doctor prior to embarking on any form of treatment, dietary regimen or supplementation.

ISBN: 0-595-18718-8

Printed in the United States of America

DEDICATION

This book is dedicated to the memory of Dr. Richard P. Murray, a man whose work in the field of biochemical research and clinical nutrition created quite a stir amidst the established medical community. Dr. Murray was a soldier on a mission—to tell the truth, exploit the untruths and to separate biochemical reality from marketing-motivated fallacies and medical approaches that only address symptoms; and even alternative healthcare practices that are, in his often-used expression "complete nonsense." I credit Dr. Murray more than any other individual with opening my eyes to seeing the reality of why people become ill and how the body depends upon food as nutritional fuel for health. Dr. Murray's intimate knowledge of biochemistry gave him the ammunition to argue why drugs, synthetic and fractionated vitamins and non-foods lead to our demise. His writings and talks were often dismissed as vicious attacks on the modern medical establishment. Yet those who could separate their egos from their true selves could see that honesty, although seemingly cruel, is the only link to reality and realization. Dr. Murray was the embodiment of the saying: "The truth will set you free, but first it will tick you off."

CONTENTS

FOREWORD

Far too much emphasis over the past fifty years in the "modern" world has been placed upon the mechanical, physical aspects of our bodies and how they work. In the wake of such scientific exploration, we seem to have lost the tradition of looking to nature and spirit as the source of our health and healing. Now, at last, many of us are rediscovering that as we become one with our food, nature and ourselves, we are empowering ourselves to transform our lives from that of "dis-ease" and discontent to one of health, vitality and inner peace. More importantly, we are learning that as intelligent, choice-making beings, we can indeed improve and change ourselves, and direct the course of our lives.

This work is a departure from the norm in that the author, Dr. Vic Shayne, shows us that the road to health and happiness is not only lined with guideposts for the maintenance of our bodies, but, more importantly, for our whole selves. This is truly the basis for the holistic healthcare movement that has gained so much deserved acceptance in recent years. In this book, Dr. Shayne has bridged the gap between our true essence and the alienation we have brought upon ourselves by our mental/ego separation from nature. He has created a union of physics and spiritual self; and gives us the inspiration to imbibe in what we can enjoy and be present in a feast with healthy foods.

Any time we are "sick" we are going to experience lowered awareness and diminished consciousness. Likewise, any time we are bogged down by lowered consciousness, we tend to ignore our physical health. Thus, with a little practice in awareness and patience for ourselves, we can enjoy life to its fullest each moment in conscious awareness. The alternative, sad but true, is to experience suffering and/or disease.

This book transcends religion and philosophy and helps us see the total or complete connection between what we think and what we are. As such, we realize that a positive approach to eating will create energy, light and vibration from our food to feed and nourish our very cells. On the other hand that feeds us, if we project a negative state of mind or being on our food while we are eating (through stress, anxiety, anger or fear of our food itself), even the healthiest of foods can fail to provide us with the nourishment that we are expecting to derive from it.

Food is our sustenance and life force, and until a book such as this one, very few realize that only when we appreciate the life force in the raw and natural states of food can we transfer and assimilate this essence into our cells. We are not always as much what we eat as what we assimilate. With all of the specific tools that Dr. Shayne bestows upon us, he takes us to the essence of the cause and effect between our actions and their consequences.

Clearly, we must love and respect ourselves to truly nurture our beings and the body temple. Dr. Shayne shares with us a vision of what it can be like to cleanse our systems, purify our minds, bodies and emotions and feel good about ourselves once again which is our true nature and given right. This book is one of the first successful attempts to bridge science, physics and nature with our own inner spirituality.

—Mark D. Smith, N.D.
University of Natural Medicine
Santa Fe, New Mexico

PREFACE

In the late 1940s, professor of medicine at Cornell University, Dr. C.W. Cavanaugh, wrote: "The fact is there is only one major disease, and that is malnutrition. All ailments and afflictions to which we may become heir are directly traceable to this major disease."

Contemporaneously, medical physician G.T. Wrench of England asserted, "The inescapable conclusion is that in a very large number of diseases, faulty food is the primary cause. The suspicion is that faulty food is the primary cause of such an overwhelming mass of disease that it may prove to be simply the primary cause of disease."

Dr. Vic Shayne's book presents more overwhelming evidence with solid documentation and demonstrates conclusively that the observations of Dr. Cavanaugh and Wrench were fifty years ahead of their time, were accurate, but possibly did not realize that the situation then, compared to the 1990s, was only a minute fraction of the declining health picture of the future.

Healthwise, we are now at the end of a civilization that is rapidly deteriorating. Hopefully, Vic Shayne's book, along with other voices in the wilderness, will help the ordinary citizen to awaken, change their dietary habits and survive a little longer with a little less suffering.

—Dr. Richard P. Murray

ACKNOWLEDGEMENTS

With the encouragement and inspiration of my good friend Gilbert Williams, D.C., I entered into this field of natural healthcare first to resolve my own health problems, then to help people understand their connection with nature and the foods they eat. I am grateful to Dr. Williams and his profound insights. Our relationship is testimony to the beneficial effects that arise when a doctor unselfishly gives of his time, resources and knowledge.

Thanks also to Mark Smith, N.D., for reviewing this book and sharing his knowledge and wisdom in the practice of natural healthcare.

I am deeply appreciative of biochemical researcher Richard P. Murray, D.C., whose pursuit of truth gives integrity to his findings and writings. Dr. Murray's intimate understanding of biochemistry and nutrition lends credibility to natural healthcare modalities. I am very grateful to him for supplying me with a wealth of carefully researched and documented resources that serve as the basis for separating fact from fiction in these days of miracle cures, misdiagnoses, (legalized) drug abuse and even "alternative" healthcare practices lacking biochemical foundation.

I also thank my friend Angi Moyer Collins who most painstakingly helped edit this work. Angi's criticisms, notes and corrections were priceless.

Lastly, I salute the many individuals who appreciate the role of nature in human health and vitality—those who understand that we are responsible not only for our own health, but also our role in maintaining the delicate balance of the internal and external environment upon which we all rely.

NUTRITION: THE MOST OVERLOOKED & UNDERRATED ASPECT OF HEALTHCARE

In the wake of marketing hype, medical and "alternative" healthcare fallacies and truisms, and a departure from nature, this book is about the most basic fact of life: health is dependent upon nutrients derived from real food, breathable air and pure water. There are also other factors, of course, upon which optimum health are built, including love, avoidance of stress, freedom of thought, exercise, reduced exposure to environmental toxins, and staying out of accidents. Some factors affecting health are fully in our control, while others are at best partially under our control. As we are heavily bombarded by a relentless stream of slanted and confusing television messages extolling the virtues of wonder drugs that supposedly make illnesses vanish by popping a pill, the TRUTH is that regaining lost health is simply not so simple. Reversing disease is a process that must be achieved biochemically and with determination and faith in nature. The building blocks of life and health are nutrients, not drugs, isolated vitamins and minerals, surgery, massage therapy, acupuncture, laser treatments, creams, lotions, or chelation therapy. The cells of the body respond to nutrients found in real, whole and natural foods. This is a fact of life which satisfies both science and common sense.

This book is about how illness is really created and how to achieve an awareness of why nutrition is essential to life; and how your choice to eat the right foods (real foods) makes the difference between health and illness. In this modern era we have been misled to believe that we may enjoy health without taking personal interest and responsibility to ensure its promotion and our longevity. And we have for too long relied on the fallacy that drugs cure disease without understanding that there's no such thing as a "drug deficiency" in the first place.

Today's choices contribute to tomorrow's state of health. This is especially pertinent in the face of today's incredible onslaught of marketing claims, corporate greed disguised as "protective measures" for the common good, persuasive (but slanted) advertising campaigns, modern medical technology and treatments, the booming alternative healthcare movement, companies selling vitamins and other supplements yielding drug-like effects, propaganda from special interest groups, and misinformation proffered by purposeful design and by unsubstantiated rumors that gel into theory and then harden into commonly accepted fact.

If we accept that we can eat anything we would like without regard to its harmful effects upon our biochemistry, then we are either headed for sickness, or we have already reached that point. On the other hand, once we realize our role in our own health by virtue of the foods we eat, our health is in our own hands (where it belongs).

YOUR DAILY DIET IS YOUR
MOST VALUABLE HEALTH ASSET

For some reason there exists a debate as to whether food has any affect on health and disease. Too many doctors definitively tell their patients, "Food has absolutely nothing to do with your being sick." (Doctors are also famous for telling their patients that food has nothing to do with overcoming an illness.) This is one of the most illogical statements that can be made, yet it is authoritatively stated again and again, adding to the confusion that exists about health and our ability to direct it.

The Merck Manual of Diagnosis & Therapy, which for the past 95 years has served to "meet the needs of general practitioners" (v)—the highly esteemed volume of *materia medica* (1435)—states, "Lack of essential dietary nutrients (e.g., from food fads, intestinal malabsorption, systemic illness, certain hereditary diseases, and anorectic states) can damage the brain, spinal cord and peripheral nerves. The common malnourished states that arise in chronic alcoholism, debilitating disease, and starvation are particularly important, since nervous system complications of these are treatable."

The Merck Manual describes an array of nutrition-related, vitamin-deficiency disorders for doctors to take note of, including chronic liver disease, cystic fibrosis, intestinal problems, amblyopia, psychosis, strokes, and so on. As biochemical researcher Dr. Richard P. Murray once said,

"Doctors who don't believe in the value of nutrition should reread their own medical school textbooks."

Most every doctor, whether M.D., D.O., D.C., Ph.D., D.D.S. or N.D., understands that to survive and be healthy, we must not only eat nutritious food, but we must also properly assimilate (use/digest) our food. At the same time, we must avoid environmental toxins and excess stress and emotional/mental negativity.

The nutrition that food offers the body marks the difference between health and disease. If most doctors admit (which they do) that vitamin C cures scurvy, that vitamin B12 cures pernicious anemia, that vitamin D prevents rickets, that calcium is needed by the bones and for healing tissue, and that without potassium the heart stops beating, then certainly they are all admitting that food has SOMETHING TO DO WITH EVERYTHING!

Food is natural, healing medicine. The consequences for not eating nutritious food is sickness, disease and premature death.

NATURE STILL HOLDS THE SECRET TO HEALTH, VITALITY & HEALING

We have entered a new and exciting era of healthcare. As a society, we have arrived at the point in which we are exploring the wonders of nature and its abundance, and how this pertains to preserving and promoting our health. Some may argue that our newfound focus on natural healthcare may be the antithesis of a world submerged (and drowning) in technology—laser beams, ultrasound, CAT scans, microsurgery, and all the rest.

It's funny how much of this antithesis is referred to as "new age" thinking or "alternative" practice. The truth is that foods, herbs and meditation have been around since the beginning of time, while chemotherapy, balloon angioplasties, bypass surgery and the like have only recently arrived on the scene. It would be more accurate to say that in the exploration of natural healthcare, we are simply moving into an age of Rediscovery. It is clear to many that the powers-that-be (large corporate interests, special interest lobbyists and established healthcare institutions) work diligently to discredit natural healthcare as a means of protecting their dominance in the practice of surgery and pharmacology.

WHAT ARE WE REDISCOVERING?

Much of what we know about natural healthcare is rooted in the traditions of ancient civilizations where the mind, body and spirit are realized to be

5

inseparable, interconnected parts of our whole selves, and balanced with the natural environment. Food and medicine are one and the same when found in a natural, unaltered and whole state. Health practitioners of all types—from medical doctors to clinical nutritionists—are rediscovering this ancient philosophy.

Such is the marvel of nature—every life form is so entwined and inter-related that to study part of the whole without considering how it affects, or is affected by, the other parts is an act of shortsightedness.

How could we consider, for example, why the leaves of a dying house plant are turning brown without considering what's going on at the root level? Is the plant getting enough water? Enough sunlight? Are the right kinds of nutrients in the soil? Certainly, we don't think that by simply trimming away the brown leaves that the plant will once again be healthy. Or do we? Oddly enough, and quite illogically, we find that in the scheme of modern medicine, this is all too frequently the approach to disease: An infected organ is cut away (removed) and the patient is sewn up and sent home. Perhaps this approach explains why more than half of all the patients of our hospitals are seeking a cure to iatrogenic causes. (Iatrogenic refers to the situation wherein today's illness is due to yesterday's unsuc-cessful "cure," or mistreatment, of the same or related illness).

As human beings, we are more than the sum total of our various bodily systems. If someone was to have a heart attack, can we assume that all a doctor has to do is repair the heart and everything else will be just fine? Of course not, especially when the patient is still left with damaged arteries, a stressful job, a bad diet or an overweight condition. Each bodily organ is connected to a system, and that system is connected to another system. (A problem with the liver, for example, may affect the health of the skin, hormones, gallbladder, nerves, cholesterol levels, and so on). Each system is influenced by a host of uncountable, interrelated factors, including the environment, thought processes, sounds, lights, marital conditions, job stress, relationship problems, food and nutrition, genetics, climate, state of consciousness, attitude, living conditions and more. All of these influences comprise the whole person and the whole health picture of the individual.

Blinded by prosperity, opportunity, social status, one-sided education and self-centeredness, too many modern-day doctors, by and large, have forgotten, ignored or never learned that their patients are WHOLE persons. This is astounding when you think about it: How can a doctor attempt to make you well without first considering and understanding the whole of who you are? It is nearly impossible, except through a stroke of blind luck and guesswork. Laboratory work may reveal certain blood abnormalities, for example, but what can this tell a doctor about what you are eating (or failing to eat) to cause or contribute to the abnormalities? Laboratory work-ups may tell the doctor about high blood sugar, elevated white blood cell count or presence of disease, but still the doctor is left with no information regarding your fears, your attitudes, marital problems, thought processes, childhood influences or most any other aspect of your WHOLE self.

Ancient societies, such as those of the Chinese, Tibetans, Indians and Native Americans, have long ago proposed that each person is intimately related to, and dependent upon, nature and spirit (that intangible aspect of the self beyond the mind and emotions). These ancient cultures continue to support the philosophy that, in body, we are not apart from nature, but rather we are *a part of* nature. They know that, *in mind*, we are creatures of habit. But they also know that, *in spirit*, we are connected to the infinite source of all life—an intangible essence that gives us feelings of love, appreciation, gratitude, upliftment, integrity, insight and intuition. It is this ability to connect with and recognize this spiritual aspect that sets us apart from other life forms, giving us a purpose for living. Perhaps most importantly, it is because we are spiritually-connected beings that we must take responsibility for our actions. We are imbued with the ability to fore-see the effects of our actions and to act intelligently and responsibly toward a good cause. In short, somewhere deep down inside we know the difference between wrong and right.

Too many individuals, religious leaders and institutions act as if mankind is here to exploit nature and ignore its laws. To have dominion over nature becomes an abusive relationship, as evidenced by the destruction of life and environment on our planet. Ironically, the figureheads of our religions have taught that on our journey through life we are destined, sooner or later, to learn to take responsibility for our every action. Each of us has the power to live up to a greater purpose—to gain the awareness that life and health is a precious gift not to be abused just because we have the power to be abusive.

THE GAME OF LIFE & HEALTH: PLAYING WITHIN THE RULES

Life is a series of choices and actions. The more conscious (aware) we are of our actions and thoughts, the greater control we have over the direction of our lives. By choosing not to think about what you eat and how your food affects your body, you are choosing ill health. Likewise, by choosing not to analyze and work on your emotional problems, you are choosing to be plagued by them as well.

LIFE HAS RULES

Ironically, most of us are involved in the game we call Life without even knowing there are rules! In the board game of Monopoly, there are rules. In society there are laws. In the physical universe there are natural laws such as gravity and inertia. Within these laws is the allowance for purposeful, willful choices borne of careful consideration. On the other hand, our ignorance of laws lays the foundation for our problems and suffering. Hence the saying, "Ignorance of the law is no excuse." If our choices are driven completely by desire or impulse rather than wisdom and insight, then suffering ensues. This is why the Dali Lama teaches that desire is the root of all suffering. We need to consider whether we desire junk food more than good health; and whether we desire destruction of our forests more than the preservation of our ozone layer and ecology.

CAUSE-AND-EFFECT RELATIONSHIP

Events in life are based on a series of cause-and-effect relationships. A specific action (cause) creates an effect (something that happens as a result of the action). Not only does this bring a sense of logic and reliability to events that occur, but it also lays the ground work for prevention of undesirable events, as well as for achievement of desired effects.

Karma is a term native to the Far East (India, China, Tibet, Japan, Korea, etc.) and has long colored the philosophical and religious teachings of far-eastern cultures. The Law of Karma teaches that for each action you take, you cause a reaction (an effect). This is a simple law whose counterpart is analogous to Sir Isaac Newton's law of physics which states that "for every action, there is an equal and opposite reaction." According to Newton's principle, if you throw a ball against a wall, it will come back to you. If it hits you in the head, it is not because the wall or ball is angry at you, but only because you set the whole event in motion and you are receiving the "fruits" of your labor. Similarly, if you eat a bag of cookies a day and you end up with a cavity in your tooth, it is not because you are being punished for your actions in the sense that your teeth are enacting revenge, but rather because you were the CAUSE of a biochemical reaction. This type of effect is the result of acting without an appreciation of the consequences—which is how most of us act in regard to most facets of our lives: We do things without being aware (or conscious) that we are creating negative results. We act in defiance of our mothers' warnings: Think before you act! Further, it is common for human beings to turn a blind eye to future suffering for a little satisfaction today.

ACTING CONSCIOUSLY

It is wonderful and fulfilling to understand and appreciate that for each of our actions we cause a reaction. With this realization, it becomes easier to avoid the pitfalls of life. With careful consideration and awareness, it becomes easier to discover how to navigate through life with fewer problems. However, having a realization about cause-and-effect relationships is not about avoiding actions *IN FEAR* of the results. Instead, it is about learning valuable lessons as a means of achieving personal growth and optimal health and vitality. When you act consciously, you become a creator instead of a reactor. If you are interested in creating greater health, then you must appreciate the fact that whatever you eat will cause a specific effect on your mind and body. With this appreciation, you gain freedom (from illness) through eating consciously. With greater awareness, you come to understand that eating the right foods is not a matter of self-denial or self-discipline, as in the typical dieting scenario, but rather an expression of your creative freedom. You are making a conscious choice to be healthy; you are planting the seeds for a healthier future. You are also generating an interest to continuously harvest more information to help gain more control over your health. This is achieved by understanding the nature of foods and their interplay with your body.

Are you free to be healthy, or are you free to BE sick ?

Forcing yourself to do anything creates an imbalance. Force goes against the "flow" of nature. If you eat healthy foods because you love yourself and you love to feel good, then you will achieve great results. If, on the other hand, you force yourself to eat healthier foods as a matter of self discipline and willful intent, then you really have not had a realization that eating healthy is the right thing to do. In this case, you are merely going through the motions, without true devotion. There is no peace of mind or personal growth that comes from force. Force does not last, because it depends solely on your willpower. Compared to the flow of the universe, willpower cannot be sustained for long without excessive wear, tear, stress and exhaustion. Which would you rather be: *disciplined* or *motivated*?

LIVE CONSCIOUSLY

Eighty-eight-year-old pioneer nutritionist and author Dr. Bernard Jensen writes, "Unless the individual educates himself in the art of conscious living and acquires rational habits and lives up to them consistently, nothing but physical and mental catastrophes can be the result."

CAUSE IS SEPARATED FROM EFFECT

The relationship between your actions and their effects may not be immediately apparent. The effects of your actions may be separated so far by time, space and conditions that it is difficult to pinpoint exactly what you may have done to make yourself sick. For instance, your sinus headache today may be the result of what you ate yesterday or even last week. Or premenstrual syndrome (PMS) can often be the result of a nutritional deficiency that only manifests itself once a month within a continuing cycle.

Doctors in the field of natural healthcare understand that the body becomes increasingly toxic over the course of time as one eats toxic foods and as one continues to be exposed to environmental poisons. As a result, in the body's effort to maintain balance and function to the best of its ability, once the body reaches certain levels of toxicity, a person may even become "used to" bad foods and not realize he/she is getting sick from eating them. Symptoms of bad nutrition may be immediate, as in a skin rash; or they may develop slowly over time, such as in the instance of heart disease, cancer, diabetes or arthritis. Add to this the factor that we are all individuals with different levels of tolerance and different inherent strengths and weaknesses. Ice cream may give me a sinus headache, while you seem only to suffer with a weight gain. But you can be sure of one thing: When you eat poorly, you do suffer whether or not you are consciously aware of the effects on your body; and whether the effects of your diet are immediately apparent or waiting in store for you in the future.

After a lifetime of "foul-nutrition," it becomes difficult to determine specifically which particular foods/nonfoods (or combinations thereof) are causing your problems. But there's hope, beginning with your awareness of your choices to avoid falling victim to the inevitable ill effects.

HOW TO ESCAPE
THE CLUTCHES OF FATE

Many people regard their illnesses as fate, or in the least, as a complete mystery. They feel helpless, victimized, trapped and unable to make significant changes in their lives because they believe that they were "dealt a hand of cards" by some divine providence determining the course of their lives. Modern medical opinion helps to promote this fatalistic belief system when our ills are blamed on genetics, bacteria, germs, viruses and mad cow disease. This kind of thinking is hopeless and depressing. It is also convenient, because it allows people to blame their state of health on their parents, upbringing, nationality, culture, bone structure, their spouse's cooking, immigrants, a busy schedule and social status. The truth is that the only thing that traps you is your own limited awareness to make conscious decisions. Making excuses is easy; making changes for the better takes a little desire and motivation—conscious effort.

The less aware you are of what is going on around you, inside you, and to you, the more you fall victim to the fate of the decisions you make (even if those decisions are unconscious).

Each of us is constantly creating. We either choose to create positively, negatively or surrender our choices to others. Disease and illness "happens" for a reason. You just have to increase your awareness to see what the reason is and what you can do about it. To do this, you must pay more attention to your body, your mind, environment, emotions and desires.

YOUR BODY IS TALKING TO YOU.

Your body communicates with you constantly. It tells you when you are hungry, thirsty, tired, nervous, energetic, cold, hot, dry, oily, tingly, injured, sore, in pain and needing to go to the bathroom. I'm sure I left a few out, but you get the idea. These are all messages coming to you from command central—your brain.

Each organ and tissue reports to your brain its relative state of health. A symptom is no more than a call for attention by your body. It may be a headache, backache, runny nose, irregular heartbeat, sinus congestion, cold sore, indigestion or aching joint.

SYMPTOMS ARE A CALL FOR HELP

How do you respond to such a call for help by your own body? Do you tell your body to "shut up and be quiet" even though it is trying desperately to communicate with you that something is amiss? Consider the fact that each time you take aspirin, antacids, or any prescription drug to suppress a symptom, you are telling your body to shut up and be quiet. You are in essence ignoring your body's call for help. When you merely treat the symptom, you allow the actual disorder or disease to worsen because you are failing to eliminate the cause of your problem. The choice is yours: to make a sensible change in your diet or lifestyle, to ignore your symptoms, or to just address the symptom and not the cause.

WHO IS IN CONTROL OF YOUR DIET?

Our pets are more or less at the mercy of our choices to feed them; and they can eat only what we put in their bowls. Yet, as human beings who are not living in captivity, we have a great bit more control over what we feed ourselves. If your teenager chooses to ingest a peanut butter sandwich, a can of cola, a box of cookies, French fries and a bag of potato chips, the effect may be acne. When this results, our society teaches that the teenager should tell his/her body to shut up and be quiet when the symptom arises. Dermatologists treat acne with antibiotics, hormones, acid baths and ultraviolet light, but this in no way addresses the ongoing destructive eating pattern. Acne is not caused by an antibiotics deficiency or a Clearisil deficiency.

When symptoms are treated instead of causes, then very little value is gained in the act. Regardless, conditioned by pharmaceutical companies, hospitals and modern medicine, most Americans are REACTIVE when it comes to their healthcare. When symptoms arise, they look for relief in surgery, injections or prescription medications and over-the-counter drugs. In the arena of alternative healthcare, too many people carry over the same mind-set by using, in similar fashion, herbs, homeopathic remedies, isolated vitamins and flower power.

Although it is an oversimplification to state that drugs are absolutely useless, there is no doubt that they are over prescribed, overused, abused, overvalued and are NOT regarded by the body as nutrients. Drugs are foreign agents that are neither natural or biochemical; they are lifeless chemicals incapable of creating life or "feeding" cells. The diseases of mankind are due to nutritional deficiencies, not drug deficiencies.

ARE YOU AWARE OF WHAT YOU EAT?

Why do you eat? Most people would answer by saying that they eat because they get hungry. The real reason why we need to eat is for nutrition. Trillions of cells in our bodies need energy to perform their myriad functions. Without nutrients, their work cannot be completed efficiently and the result—the effect—is dis-ease.

Now let's take a look at some of the common foods in the America diet and relate them to disease. First, consider the "food groups." Where did the notion of outlining so-called basic dietary food groups (dairy, wheat, vegetables, meat, etc.) come from? It's hard to say. However, one gets the sneaking suspicion that the cereal, beef, poultry and dairy industries, along with those companies specializing in the sale and marketing of devitalized foods had their hands in the ballot box. An ongoing public relations and advertising and marketing campaign by these groups has led us to believe that their meat and dairy products are essential to your health, which is highly debatable. Millions of people suffer with mucus congestion, sinus headaches, weight gain, severe gas and breathing problems by consuming dairy products. Some doctors such as cardiologist Dean Ornish, M.D., have related red meat consumption to heart disease. Yet the marketing messages put out by dietitians' associations and large corporations mislead people into accepting that we all share the same dietary needs and biochemical requirements. The truth is that each of our particular nutritional needs are different from anyone else's.

The food pyramid and food group concepts are attempts to make a general issue out of a very complex and individualistic matter. So let's forget about thinking about foods in groups because this takes our minds off of the real problem at hand—Most of the foods in the typical American diet are nutritionally inadequate, and the effect from eating these non-foods results in nutritional deficiencies and disease. To take this one step further, most of what we now call food is really not food at all, but rather lifeless, chemicalized concoctions that threaten health and life.

ARE YOU EATING REAL FOOD?
—OR SUFFERING FROM 'FOUL-NUTRITION'?

Major food manufacturers produce items that should not even be called "food." The typical food market/grocery store is jam-packed with items that contain a wide array of substances foreign to, and harmful to, the body. So why do people eat them?

Long before I learned the difference between a food and a chemical concoction, I used to choose foods, like most Americans, based on whether they tasted good to me. I took for granted that I was protected by the government, the FDA and other groups who I thought made sure that all the food sold in this country and in restaurants was safe enough to eat. I was dead wrong. The truth is that today's foods contain substances that are making most of our population sick. Not only do they fail to provide us with the basic building blocks of life, including vitamins, minerals, trace elements, good fats, co-enzymes, enzymes, amino acids, chlorophyll, fiber, proteins and other nutrients, but they are also filled with dangerous constituents.

Modern grocery store foods are loaded with chemicals and toxins—pesticide residues, solvent residues, synthetic fertilizers, preservatives, additives, artificial sweeteners, refined sugars, hydrogenated oils, artificial flavors, emulsifiers, dyes, hormones and synthetic vitamins (so-called "enriched"). Having these non-foods in your diet over the course of time (especially over the course of a lifetime) will take their toll. They will cause disease; it's only a matter of time. If you are not getting your nutrition from the foods you eat, then your body cannot function as it was designed—it begins to break down, even before symptoms or disease become apparent. When you eat foods containing "non-food" ingredients, you are the effect of a double-whammy. First, you are starving your body of needed nutrients; and, secondly, adding insult to injury, you are being poisoned at the same time.

Biochemical researcher Dr. Richard P. Murray said, "Americans may be the MOST fed people on earth, but certainly not the BEST fed."

READ THE LABELS!

Janet Tubbs, author of *If You Can't Pronounce It, Don't Eat It!*, says it all in the title of her book. Although we all expect to feed our bodies for the sake of health, most people who shop in grocery stores do not read carefully the labels on their food packages. It doesn't take an Einstein to understand that the contents of refined foods (typical grocery store foods) are not native to the human biochemistry. You will not find Yellow Dye #5 on a tree; MSG is not found in roots; and you won't find partially hydrogenated oils in any vegetable or grain on Earth. There's no such thing as a synthetic vitamin in any of the millions of species of plants; NO vitamin, including vitamin C ascorbic acid, EVER exists alone (by itself, in isolation) in a real food. These chemicals should not be in the diet. So, why do people eat them?

There are nine main reasons why you may eat foods that are refined and full of chemicals:

1. You may not read labels on food packages;
2. You may trust food manufacturers to only put wholesome, nutritious ingredients in their products;

3. You may trust the government to protect you from food manufac-turers responsible for adding non-nutritious, unhealthy ingredients to their products;

4. You may eat foods based on their taste, texture, color and smell rather than their nutritional quality;

5. You may believe that food manufacturers and their commercial messages are truthful. You may be under the illusion (or confusion) that their products are good for you;

6. You may find that REAL foods are more expensive and you choose to eat non-foods based on financial concerns;

7. Perhaps you have never thought about this matter before because no one ever brought it to your attention;

8. You may be aware that your diet consists of non-foods, but you are too lazy to make a change; or

9. You may be aware of your diet of non-foods, but you believe they will not adversely affect your health.

REFINED FOODS

Refined foods are foods that have been altered from their original, natu-ral state to such a degree that they become devitalized (lifeless) and destructive in the human body. Real foods contain vitamins, enzymes and other life-supporting properties. Food manufacturers change real foods into non-foods/refined foods by heating, chemical alteration and infusion, milling, and removing (or altering) portions that easily spoil. As a result, refined foods, such as refined wheat and/or refined sugars used for cereals, breads, cakes, condiments, etc., are not accepted or usable by our cells as nutrients. In fact, these refined foods cause problems ranging from low blood sugar symptoms to chronic fatigue, from obesity to diabetes, from hormonal imbalances to liver disease, and from headaches to PMS. The vitamins, proteins, essential fats and enzymes in foods are most often destroyed or changed into health-damaging substances by the time foods have undergone the refining process.

You may ask: Why do food manufacturers refine perfectly good foods? The answer is economics. Knowing that natural oils in foods spoil (as they are designed to do by nature), food manufacturers alter or remove these oils to give foods longer shelf life and to control taste. It is cheaper to refine foods than to bring them to the grocery store in their original state only to have them spoil. And, refined foods can be made more attractive with additives, preservatives, emulsifiers and flavor enhancers. With enough chemical additives, cardboard can be made to taste good. While all of this is great for food manufacturers and their bulging pocketbooks, it is disastrous for human beings whose cells rely on real food for energy, immunity, mental acuity, mobility, growth, repair and maintenance.

We are now at a critical juncture in our history where entire generations have been brought up on refined, toxic foods without ever having consumed sufficient quantities of REAL foods as found in nature. The incidence of disease in this country continues to escalate as a result of this "foul-nutrition" and malnutrition. Children are being brought up on breakfast cereals that are not only devoid of nutrition, but are actually candy disguised as food. The vitamins with which these cereals have been "enriched" are no more than synthetic chemicals injected to pacify the public's confused concern for what it perceives is proper nutrition. (We will address vitamin-enriched foods in a subsequent chapter.)

In addition to malnutrition from non-food diets, one of the greatest threats to human health is toxic substances, including pesticides, which are ingested into the body through so-called foods.

According to a new analysis of federal data by the Environmental Working Group (EWG), Washington, DC, "Every day, 1 million American children age 5 and under consume unsafe levels of a class of pesticides that can harm the developing brain and nervous system." The EWG's report, *Overexposed: Organophosphate Insecticides in Children's Food*, states that peaches, apples, pears and grapes are the most common sources of exposure to unsafe levels of organophosphate pesticides (OPs) for young children. The report says the solution is not for infants, children and pregnant women to eat fewer fruits and vegetables, but to rid these otherwise healthful foods of the most dangerous pesticides. EWG vice president for research Richard Wiles, lead author of this study, suggests: "Kids should be able to eat a diet rich in fruits and vegetables without risking brain or nerve damage."

The above report was in response to the Food Quality Protection Act, passed unanimously by Congress in 1996, that required all pesticides to be "safe" for infants and children. (Unfortunately, this requirement has never been met. In fact, logically speaking, how can a pesticide ever be safe considering that pesticides are designed to kill living organisms?). The law further stipulated that combined exposures to pesticides be considered when setting safety standards.

Wiles stated, "This study shows that every day, hundreds of thousands of children receive unsafe exposures, at precisely the age when they are most vulnerable to long- and short-term brain and nervous system damage."

According to Environmental Working Group:

> The EWG report was based on more than 80,000 samples of food tested by the U.S. Department of Agriculture and the Food and Drug Administration (FDA), and dietary records for more than 4,000 children collected by the USDA. The foods that cause the most children age 5 and under to exceed a safe daily dose of OP pesticides are apples, peaches and grapes. Almost one-fourth of the times a young child eats a peach, that child is consuming an unsafe level of OP pesticides. About one apple in eight will expose a child to an unsafe dose.

For infants 6 to 12 months old, commercial baby food is the dominant source of unsafe levels of pesticides (as well as other chemicals) in food. Every day, about 77,000 infants are exposed to unsafe levels through eating baby food preparations of apple juice, apple sauce, pears and peaches.

"The point is not that parents should avoid feeding baby food to their children, the point is that pesticides in baby food are not safe for babies. Baby food should not have any pesticides in it at all. We think if you ask parents, they will agree," said Wiles. "In the meantime, organic baby food provides parents with an added measure of safety," Wiles added.

Environmental Working Group states:

> Estimates of the number of children at risk are conservative not only because kids are also exposed to pesticides sprayed in their homes, schools and day care centers, but because the EPA's current standards are based on levels considered safe for adults. The EWG study estimates that if the EPA set standards to comply with the Food Quality Protection Act, which requires an additional ten-fold margin of safety, as many as 3.6 million children aged 6 months to 5 years could be considered at risk.

"There is no scientific justification for allowing levels of pesticides in food that put more than one million children at risk each day," said Kert Davies, co-author of the report.

The study found that of the 13 OP pesticides found in or on food by the USDA and FDA, most of the risk to children comes from five chemicals: methyl parathion, dimethoate, chlorpyrifos, pirimiphos methyl and azinphos methyl. The report urges that these five pesticides be banned immediately for all agricultural use, and also recommends:

• A ban on all home and other structural use of OP pesticides.
• A ban on all OP pesticides on commodities that end up in baby food.
• Safety standards for all OP pesticides must be set at levels that are safe for infants and children.

Acres, USA (February 2001) reported:

> A study in the journal *Cancer* shows that pesticide exposure appears to increase the risk of a certain type of cancer in children—possibly as much as sevenfold. The amount of pesticides a child is exposed to—both prenatally and

postnatally—and that child's chances of developing non-Hodgkin's lymphoma, a cancer that arises in the lymphatic system, are at the base of the study. Experts agree these findings are preliminary and require more detailed research, "But there's pretty good evidence here," said Brad H. Pollock, Ph.D., m.P.H., interim chair of the department of health policy and epidemiology at the University of Florida College of Medicine…The data from this study should serve as a starting point for further research, including looking at the genetic changes caused by pesticides and identifying the specific cancer-causing substances in the pesticides.

Once you begin to eat refined foods and foods laden with toxic chemicals (which nowadays is from the point of birth!), not only is your body starving for real nutrition, but it is at the same time becoming depleted of health. The situation is analogous to putting fake money into your bank account while taking real money out to meet your obligations. Eventually you reach bankruptcy—ill health.

The secret to safe food consumption is to begin by reading labels. If names of chemicals appear on your food labels, you should not eat the food. For instance, a peanut butter label should state "peanuts and salt." No other ingredients necessary. What does your label state? Chemicals, whether pesticides, emulsifiers or dyes, do not belong in foods.

ARE WE BEING ATTACKED BY GERMS, OR JUST POISONING OURSELVES?

Why are scientists and doctors admittedly losing the war on cancer? Why does the incidence of cancer continue to rise? Certainly, it's not because we lack enough drugs in our modern medical arsenal! (Remember that no one gets sick because of a drug deficiency.) Disease results from a body under assault. When people eat foods laden with pesticides meant to kill living organisms (that's the role of a pesticide!), then they become poisoned and ill. The poisoning may take a long time to notice, but just the same, it takes place. In addition to environmental poisons, today's supermarket foods are supply lines of dangerous chemicals that cannot be used by—and are destroying—the human body.

People who have been subsisting on a diet of REAL foods—organically grown fruits, vegetables, grains, nuts and seeds and organically-raised meats—are often able to taste the chemicals in non-foods as if they are biting into a bar of soap. Sadly, however, most people weaned on the American fare are so used to eating foods filled with chemicals that they don't even taste them. It's true that food manufacturers work very hard to create tasty chemical concoctions, but the unspoiled, healthy eater can often detect the difference.

In *The Safe Shopper's Bible*, author David Steinman writes,

Consumers today want to make intelligent, informed shopping decisions. Until now, however, most have been shopping in the dark. They receive little guidance from food producers and product manufacturers, whose advertising and labeling are too often misleading and not objective sources of information. Government also offers little guidance. Indeed, while many local, state and federal government agencies are entrusted with protection of the public health, most have failed to assure consumers they are being adequately protected, or that they are being provided with full, if any, label disclosure of carcinogenic (i.e., cancer-causing), neurotoxic (i.e., causing damage to the nervous system), and reproductive effects, including teratogenic (i.e., birth defect-causing) chemicals in their foods and household products.

It is believed by a growing number of natural healthcare practitioners that, more often than not, what the modern medical community labels as the flu or a viral infection or even a 24-hour-bug is in reality the body's reaction to toxic poisoning or exposure to extreme temperature changes. Poisonous substances may, for example, be emitted from an industrial accident, nuclear spills, paint and chemical fumes, chemical waste dumping or pesticide spraying and affect a specific geographic location. For the next several days, a "mysterious" outbreak of illness may become apparent, causing fever, bone chill, aching muscles, runny nose, sinus pain, etc. The illness is blamed on a contagious disease (viral or bacterial), but the REAL cause is the chemical exposure; and the symptoms are merely the body's reaction to the assault. Such poisoning is epidemic, with toxic substances now attacking us in foods, the air, the water, the soil and anywhere pesticides or chemicals are used carelessly—in schools, at home, in parks and recreation sites, in public restrooms, in restaurants, at the office, in public buildings, etc. What is blamed on a virus or on bacteria is often really just chemical poisoning. Usually, the news media will help promote the epidemic by scaring the general public out of its wits while, at the same time, drumming up business for antibiotics waiting at the ready.

The next time you or a family member "catches cold," think about how the illness may have been caused by exposure to temperature changes (running out in the cold weather without enough clothing), or exposure to chemicals in the environment (paint fumes, pesticide fumes, industrial spills, etc.). The symptoms of a body under attack by chemicals is the same as that of the "flu" or a cold, including fever, runny nose, bowel problems, cramps, chills, fatigue, headache, abnormal heartbeat, etc.

NATURE'S FOOD IS OUR MEDICINE: NOBODY GETS SICK DUE TO A DRUG DEFICIENCY!

In ancient days, when illness struck, people reached for a particular food or herbal substance which would make the sickness go away. Somehow, in our progression (or regression?) through history, our society has lost sight of the healing properties of foods, herbs, sunshine, outdoor air, colors, sounds, meditation, and so forth. Yet all of these things are natural, just like us. But somewhere along the line, it was decided by the powers that be that when we get sick we should turn to drugs, surgery and injections for healing. (Although I am not suggesting that none of these modern forms of healthcare have a place in the world, I do feel that they deserve a much smaller role).

Drugs do not build new tissue; this is nature's task. Drugs tend to alleviate many symptoms, including swelling, headaches, backaches, fevers, pain, blockages, bleeding, blood clots, high blood pressure, congestion and so forth, yet, as chemicals, they always create a side effect in the body. This is important to remember in the scheme of things, because drug use does not eliminate the *cause* of an illness, only (sometimes) the effect. You can consume artificial sweeteners in your favorite soda all day long, but when you have to take an aspirin for the resulting headache, you can be guaranteed that this drug will have no power to stop you from ever drinking diet sodas again. If the aspirin takes your headache away, don't be misled into thinking that your body is not still suffering from the artificial sweeteners just because your senses have been too dulled to notice anymore.

At one time in history, medicines were derived solely from plants and animals, not synthetic/artificial chemicals. Synthetic drugs are unnatural. Drugs which are made of chemicals such as coal tar and laboratory compounds are seen by the body as poisons—foreign invaders. This has been proven by the body's response to such substances. When drugs, including synthetic vitamins, enter the bloodstream, the body acts as if it is being attacked, and it tries to rid itself of the chemicals by stimulating white blood cell activity, creating inflammation, speeding up the heart rate, presenting other symptoms (as side effects) and/or attempting to direct the offending substances out of the body (through kidneys, bowels, lungs and skin).

If the body does not eliminate all of a drug (or any toxic substance for that matter), its residues are deposited in the tissues and go to work creating new problems for the body. If you have used antibiotics, for example, it is not uncommon for your bowel to become overrun by "unfriendly bacteria" that was once kept in check by "friendly" bacteria destroyed by the antibiotics.

The rising to prominence of drugs—also referred to as *pharmaceuticals*— is directly related to politics, marketing and economics. Natural plant foods such as lemons, bananas, carrots, celery, beets and chlorophyll foods, for example, cannot be patented for their medicinal value. However, stronger compounds created from chemicals can indeed be patented and price-controlled. With a little creative marketing, pharmaceutical manufacturers, through the vehicle of modern medical doctors, have cornered the market on modern healthcare in which drug sales are measured in the billions of dollars annually. Modern society has grown so removed from the concept of natural healthcare that it has succumbed to the fear of illness given to us in high dosages by those who control the drugs, hospitals, insurance companies and treatment centers. As a society, we do not trust nature because we have been taught/ brainwashed to accept as truth the illusion that good health is a matter of getting rid of our symptoms and that drugs cure disease.

SYMPTOMS OF DISEASE ARE EFFECTS, NOT CAUSES

Symptoms of disease are only effects, and not causes. Most symptoms are merely signs that the body is at work trying to recover from some assault. Most notably, the body goes through a wondrous biochemical system of inflammation and repair that is usually treated by modern medicine as the disease itself!

> Inflammation is a process by which the body's white blood cells and chemicals protect our bodies from infection by foreign substances…When inflammation occurs, chemicals from the body's white blood cells are released into the blood or affected tissues to protect your body from foreign substances. This release of chemicals increases the blood flow to the area of injury or infection, and may result in redness and warmth. Some of the chemicals cause a leak of fluid into the tissues, resulting in swelling. This protective process may stimulate nerves and cause pain. (Cleveland Clinic, Department of Rheumatic and Immunologic Diseases; OnHealth Network Company; November 1999)

Elaborating, leading herbalist David Hoffman writes:

> Inflammation, a process unpleasantly familiar to everyone, occurs in response to a range of traumas from sunburn and wounds, to infection and auto-immune conditions. Whatever the cause, this process is basically the same…It is characterized by four physical signs; warmth, redness, swelling, and pain. Warmth and redness result from dilation of the small blood vessels in the injured area and increased local blood flow…The biochemistry and medical pathology

of this complex process [of inflammation] can often subtly imply that chemistry is the medical answer. Plants as whole medicines will reduce and soothe much inflammation whether we know the biochemistry or not. A review of recent studies show much confirmation about the efficacy of traditional remedies. (David L. Hoffman, M.N.I.M.H. *Inflammation and Arthritis*)

If drugs interfere with the process of inflammation as the body is trying to heal itself, there may not be complete repair. Signs (symptoms) of the biochemical process of inflammation and repair include swelling, redness, soreness, pus, mucus secretion, excess phlegm, bacteria (which engulf dead cells caused by the underlying disease), and heat (temperature increase, including localized and whole-body fever). Therefore, when substances (including drugs, herbs, synthetic vitamins, etc.) are used solely to alleviate these symptoms, you can see that the body's work is being short-circuited.

FOODS THAT HEAL

We know that foods can heal and that they can be good for us, but which foods do what? A complete list of all the healing factors in food as well as all of the diseases from which people suffer is nigh impossible to create. However, the following are examples of specific whole and unadulterated/ unprocessed foods that can be used to support specific body systems. Keep in mind that we are all individuals—all different—with different body types, genetic make-up, lifestyles, attitudes, and biochemical needs. What's good for you may not necessarily be needed by your cousin Bruno; and what aggravates your Aunt Tootsie's sinuses may actually be your own best friend...

SKIN: apples, rice bran, whole oats, onions, almonds, salmon, walnuts, fish, cod liver oil.

BONES: green leafy vegetables, cabbage, coconut, kelp, raw cheese and raw milk (unpasteurized), sesame seeds, veal bone meal.

HEART: whole wheat and other whole grains, especially germ (for vitamin B factors), figs, beets, bananas, potatoes, grapes, olives, green leafy vegetables, avocados, hawthorn berries, brown rice, bran, tomatoes, egg yolk.

BLOOD: black cherries, green vegetables, chlorophyll foods (greens), raisins, asparagus, onions, garlic, fish, egg yolk, parsley, raw goats milk, cucumbers, leeks, currants, burdock root, cabbage, chickweed, sesame seed butter (tahini).

RESPIRATORY TRACT: onions, garlic, seeds, fish, beets, almond milk (raw), greens, lemons, oranges, grapefruits, tomatoes, cod liver oil.

KIDNEYS: non-chlorinated water, beets, watermelon, seed drinks, real cranberry juice.

BOWELS: fresh fruits, vegetables, bran, flaxseed, water, blackberry, molasses.

BRAIN & NERVES: brown (unrefined) rice, fish, broccoli, almonds, raw egg yolk, nuts, seeds, artichoke, seafood, flaxseed oil.

MUSCLES: green leafy vegetables, meat, bananas, figs, figs, water.

JOINTS: raw goat milk, green leafy vegetables, flaxseed oil, water, celery, cucumber, parsley, strawberries, sesame seeds, currants, raw cane juice.

EYES: carrots, dandelion greens, eyebright, beets, cod liver oil.

LIVER: beets, carrots, fish, cod liver oil, tomatoes, tomato juice, artichoke, bayberry bark tea, chicory tea, parsley, milk thistle, liver from organically-raised cattle.

STOMACH: raw goat milk, celery, cucumber, strawberries.

Considering the amounts of toxic sprays and food irradiation used in and on most store-bought foods, fresh organically grown foods (by reliable growers with integrity) are the recommended alternative. Often people will report an adverse reaction from eating certain raw fruits or vegetables, yet find no difficulty at all with their organically grown counterparts. Pesticide and synthetic fertilizer residues may be blamed for adverse reactions in many cases rather than the food itself. So-called food "allergies" are very frequently blamed for sore throats, swollen gums, watery eyes and skin eruptions that occur after eating chemical-laced foods or breathing pesticide vapors coming in through your bedroom window. Pesticides are poisons designed to kill living beings or render them sterile. Although we are not insects, it is foolish to believe that such poisons (especially as they accumulate in our daily diet) do not adversely affect us as well. Before claiming that you are the hopeless effect of allergies, try an elimination diet, ridding your diet of pesticides and other offensive chemicals that are known to cause reactions commonly called "allergies."

FOOD COMBINING ISSUES:
EASING DIGESTION
& SIMPLIFYING THE DIET

Much has been written about the subject of Food Combining over the past several years, including works by Harvey and Marilyn Diamond, authors of *Fit for Life*, and a very complicated book called *Food Combining Made Easy*, by Dr. Herbert Shelton. If you are an avid reader of popular books on natural healthcare, then perhaps you are already familiar with food combining, a theory that when one mixes various foods at the same time in the same meal, the results are often poor digestion and other complications. The "rules" of food combining were created based on the theory that certain foods such as fruits, should never be consumed with certain other foods such as meats because the results will be indigestion, "putrefaction," the build-up of poisons in the digestive tract, and other unpleasant side effects.

As a clinical nutritionist, I have come to one conclusion that can be said about everybody: None of us are alike. In relation to food combining issues, it can be said that many individuals enjoy great benefits by simplifying their diets. If indigestion, bloating, overweight or other bad side effects from eating are common to you, then there is certainly no harm in giving food combining a try. Here is a simple chart to show you the basics of food combining:

In one meal, do not combine:
Meats with fruits;
Vegetables with fruits;
Meats with starches (such as rice or potatoes);
Milk (and other dairy) with meats.

THE THEORY BEHIND FOOD COMBINING

Note that the word "theory" is used to describe the issue of food combining because, although this practice may aid in digestion, experts are divided whether it has merit in the world of physiology. Pundits of food combining tell us that certain foods use specific enzymes to break them down in the process of digestion. This is true—carbohydrates are broken down by bodily enzymes such as amylase, while fats use enzymes such as lipase, and proteins are broken down by enzymes such as protease. Further, it is said that each type of enzyme works only in a certain environment—either alkaline or acid. This is also true. For instance, when you eat a starchy vegetable like a potato, the enzyme used to break it down (amylase) does not function in an acid environment like the stomach. Instead, it is digested in the mouth and in the small intestine. On the other hand, meat, being a protein food, is digested in an acid environment in the stomach, but not in an alkaline environment like the mouth or small intestine.

If you are with me so far, you may grasp the logic behind food combining which states that, when you eat meat and a potato in the same meal, the body cannot adequately break down both of these substances because they need different environments in which to do their work: the potato needs alkalinity and the meat needs acidity. The result, say theorists, is indigestion of some sort. Die-hard food combining practitioners will swear that poor food combining is the cause of numerous diseases.

ANOTHER VIEWPOINT

Why is food combining only a theory? The hitch is this: many natural, whole foods contain all three types of nutrients: proteins, carbohydrates and fats. For example, a pea or a bean may be known as a starch vegetable, but it also contains protein and fat. Similarly speaking, a walnut contains fat, proteins and carbohydrates. There is no way to avoid the three types of nutrients in one single whole, natural food. (Nor would you want to, because the body needs all three).

Many nutritionists claim that our bodies have an innate intelligence that allows them to know what kind of food is put into them and how to break the food down for digestion, even with the presence of carbohydrates, fats and proteins in the same food. (The food must be natural—we are not talking about artificial foods or chemical concoctions.) When a natural food is introduced into your body, it adjusts the timing and quantity of digestive enzymes to that particular food substance. In this way, for example, your body is able to break down a bean to utilize its inherent proteins, carbohydrates and fats.

According to some healthcare "experts," on the other hand, the issue of food combining is way overblown, with exaggerated reported results not befitting the science of physiology. However, the reader may be assured that there is no harm adhering to food combining rules; and, in fact, because most people eat poorly, proper food combining may be just what the doctor ordered to enhance and simplify digestion. After all, digestion is one of the most underestimated aspects of health, commonly overlooked by doctors treating diseased patients. Digestion is the process whereby we absorb and utilize nutrients from the foods we eat; so to enhance this process is to benefit the entire body and all of its systems.

A SEPARATE ISSUE ALTOGETHER

If you ingest (eat) an UNNATURAL mixture of foods (including processed foods, heated oils, pesticide residues, refined sugars, steroids and hormones, food additives, dyes and preservatives), your body does not respond well to their assault. This, however, is due more to the fact that these are "non-foods" rather than because you are not following the rules of food combining. Therefore, instead of being concerned with avoiding specific combinations of foods in the same meal, it would be more apropos to first avoid consuming devitalized, overcooked, processed, refined and unnatural foods. Food combining rules aside, any nonfood may potentially wreak havoc on digestion. The real issue here is NOT only whether such substances will be digested, but rather that such non-foods fail to offer you real nutrition—and even worse, that they are making you ill.

YOU DECIDE FOR YOURSELF

With all of what has been written here about food combining, it seems that you need to make up your own mind by experimentation. If you feel better by not combining certain groups of foods with other groups, then by all means, do that which makes you healthiest. If you suffer from digestive problems, or you are trying to get to the bottom of what foods cause you the most distress, then food combining may be a perfect way for you to isolate the cause of a problem by simplifying your diet.

DISEASE BEGINS IN
THE FOOD STORE
(& IS PREPARED IN THE KITCHEN)

The real purpose for eating is to bring nutrients into your body and thereby feed your cells those substances needed for growth, repair, maintenance, immunity, digestion, waste disposal, mobility, etc. This is the REAL purpose for eating, but something has gone amiss! Although the human body thrives on whole, fresh, unaltered, natural foods, the Great American Diet has become an abomination of chemical concoctions that are so far removed from having any food value that we have become a very sick nation. Due to our industrialization and influence, we have brought the wonders of the Great American Diet to other parts of the world as well. Now Japan, China, and all of Europe are partaking in our foul-nutrition gleaned from chemicals in the diet and fast food restaurants.

While certain foods may be tasty, your body cannot live in health when it subsists on a diet of hamburgers, fries, milk shakes, ham and cheese sandwiches basted with hydrogenated mayonnaise on refined bread, soft drinks, and a bag of chips. Pardon me, I seem to have omitted two scoops of ice cream bathed in chocolate sauce for dessert.

FACE THE FACT: AMERICAN DIETS ARE TOXIC

If American manufacturers could win a truly deserving award in the food industry, it would be in the category of The Prettiest Packaging, with a runner-up award of The Best Advertising Sales Job. People are so enamored with colorful package designs and hip TV ads that they fail to actually read the labels to know what they are about to put into their bodies. By distracting people from the questionable and unsafe ingredients in their products while focusing on relatively unimportant selling points such as taste, modern day food manufacturers are engaging in a sophisticated, albeit clever, sleight of hand. The greatest advice to give anyone is to read labels carefully. Know what you are eating. Look beyond the illusion and discover what's really in that brightly colored box diverting your attention with those cute little cartoon characters munching on some crunchy cookies.

Compared to the rest of the population, Baby Boomers are less likely to read food labels, less likely to worry about serving foods with "harmful" ingredients, and less likely to diet, according to a report released by The NPD Group's National Eating Trends Service. The Report on Eating Patterns of Baby Boomers examines the eating habits of the 78 million consumers born between 1946 and 1964 who represent 30% of the population and the largest consumer group in the U.S. today. According to the report, only 29% of Baby Boomers surveyed read food labels frequently, compared to 38% of the rest of the population. Like most consumers, Boomers' number one dietary concern is fat intake. However, they are less concerned about fat than the average consumer. Four out of ten Boomers say they try to avoid it, compared to five out of ten consumers among the total population. Baby Boomers are also less concerned about cholesterol, salt, additives, preservatives, sugar and caffeine....

While the number of meals eaten at home by the average American has remained constant since 1986, Baby Boomers are eating in [at home] less frequently. NPD's survey found that Americans between the ages of 29 and 47 have increased their use of restaurants by about 8% since 1986. In 1993, they spent 23% more than the average individual on restaurant dining. (Source: The NPD Group's National Eating Trends Service. The Report on Eating Patterns of Baby Boomers)

According to the above survey, nearly three out of four of baby boomers' restaurant meals were purchased at a fast food restaurant.

WHAT ARE THEY TRYING TO SELL US?

Take time to listen—to become aware of—what television advertising is trying to get you to hear. One ad for a children's cereal boldly states: "Who cares what's in it as long as it tastes good!" Another ad advises the viewer to "smooth out" their stressful day with a candy bar.

Today's food is also sold on its convenience: "Just pop it in the microwave!" (Years before, they used to say "Just pop it in the toaster!") TV dinners offer quite an amusing presentation: they are packaged in aluminum, contain all sorts of chemicals, preservatives and additives, contain no living food and are further assaulted by even more cooking in the oven. Roadkill is not as dead as most fast foods!

WHAT'S REALLY IN THE "FOOD"?

The substances we call "food" these days has little or no right to be called "food." The word "food" should be reserved for nutritious substances that nourish our bodies and contain no harmful, toxic substances. A diet full of non-foods sentences the eater to something worse than malnutrition; it's called "foul-nutrition."

How foul is America's nutrition? If you dropped in for a visit to Earth from another planet (much more mentally evolved than our own), you would be dumbfounded to discover what people eat. Hovering over a backyard barbecue you could observe a family sharing great times and joyous laughter while consuming the following: A hamburger (laced with hormones, steroids, antibiotics and other chemicals) grilled until scorched over a high flame (altering the chemistry of the meat's fat and protein and covering it with soot), placed upon a white-flour bun enriched with synthetic vitamins, refined flour, refined sugars and chemical preservatives, topped with refined-sugar-drenched ketchup and served up with potatoes fried in indigestible oils with a dessert comprised of food dyes, refined sugars, etc. Can the human body actually subsist on these non-foods? No, it eventually breaks down and fails to function as intended from the pattern of assault. Next comes a trip to the doctor wherein the patient is told that he has "contracted" a disease for which the treatment is drugs, surgery or injections. More often than not, the doctor himself shares the same type of diet that brings his patient to him for help.

The solution? It is fully possible to enjoy a hamburger lunch with all the trimmings using higher quality ingredients—ketchup without refined sugar, organic/free-range beef cooked only until pink, organic potatoes lightly baked, whole wheat/chemical-free buns and natural desserts. Still delicious and fun, but minus the poisons and nutrient-robbing substances.

WHO'S MINDING THE MINT?
CREATING CANCER BY DEFAULT

Consumers are misled to believe they are protected by government agencies from having toxic substances in their foods and personal care products. Somehow—and you can blame it on politics, economics or greed—government agencies have done little to protect us from industrial giants who are more interested in profits than public health.

David Steinman and Samuel S. Epstein, M.D., in their book *The Safe Shopper's Bible* (page 4), write:

The U.S. Food and Drug Administration (FDA)…is responsible for ensuring the safety of foods, cosmetics, prescription and over-the-counter drugs. Yet, FDA officials have consistently trivialized the risk of pesticides, industrial chemicals, food additives and animal drugs added to the food supply, and its enforcement record has been strongly criticized. Furthermore, while the FDA has initiated label disclosure of the nutritional content of foods, it has completely failed to put into place any program that would disclose chemicals applied to foods that cause cancer, nervous system damage and birth defects. Put another way, the FDA insists on labeling foods for cholesterol, but not for carcinogens [cancer-causing agents].

Even when foods are approved by government agencies to contain "acceptable levels" of various chemicals and poisons, there is NO CONSIDERATION given for the total amounts any one consumer may ingest in the course of a day. Nor is there any consideration for the way various combinations of chemicals and toxins interact with one another once they are inside your body. Therefore, of more danger than one isolated "acceptable" chemical posing "negligible risk," when you consume many different "food" products which comprise your daily diet, you are more than likely taking in more poisons than your body can eliminate.

John Steinman writes:

Based on the Environmental Protection Agency's (EPA) estimates, residues of 60 carcinogenic [cancer-causing] pesticides on thirty foods that may be eaten in just one day would result in about 64,000 excess cancers a year, more than 10 percent of all current cancer deaths. Furthermore, the EPA's estimates ignore the following exposures: undisclosed inert carcinogenic pesticide ingredients, other carcinogens in food, notably color additives; residues of hormonal animal feed additives in beef; and other chemical and radioactive carcinogens not only in food, but also in air, water and the workplace. EPA estimates also ignore unpredictable synergistic interactions from these multiple exposures, especially the cancer-accelerating effects among radiation, pesticides and hormones.

Judith DeCava, *Conquering Cancer: Illusions or Solutions?* (p.139-141), writes:

Unfortunately, when it comes to potentially harmful food additives, we take the risk while the food processors take the benefits." How much exposure to a carcinogen does it take to initiate cancer? No one knows for certain. The average annual American diet includes at least 5,000 artificial food additives.

...Some 2,100 chemical compounds have been "officially" detected in U.S. drinking water. Of these, about 190 are known or suspected to be dangerous. Many of the remaining compounds have not been adequately studied....The majority of food additives are used to enhance "consumer acceptability"—to feed illusions, make foods look fresh or look like advertisers' expectations, and to have "keeping" quality (shelf life). In other words, they are used for profit. Foods are thus bright in color, unblemished and embalmed. For "standard" foods (over 300 which do not have to list ingredients), the manufacturer can choose among many alternative standard chemicals, and only if he/she substitutes or adds a nonstandard chemical or uses Yellow No. 5, must the fact be listed on the label. The law does not require that chemicals added in small amounts during processing—even if they may be possible or probable carcinogens—be stated on the label.... Cancer may take years to develop, particularly with the accumulation of tiny and consistent amounts of a toxin. It is also not known how additives interact with each other and/or with the 63,000 other chemicals in common use today.

IF IT'S NOT REAL FOOD,
THEN WHY EAT IT?

The non-foods that should be avoided include ALL non-foods. If it's not a real food, why eat it? Real foods are actually tastier than nonfoods, not to mention the fact that they don't destroy your health. Once you are on a diet of real foods, nonfoods begin to taste like the chemicals of which they are made. Here's some inside information on commonly consumed nonfoods...

MILK

Avoid drinking nonorganic, pasteurized milk and dairy products. Milk (in its uncooked, unpasteurized form) is a substance primarily for the young. Thanks (or no thanks) to the marketing efforts of our dairy industry, we have come to believe that milk is essential in the human diet. After weaning, no other animal to be found in nature (and that covers about all of us), has milk in its diet. Despite this fact, however, milk is still potentially a good source of nutrition, except as it is found in most grocery stores.

With consistent advertising and marketing, the dairy industry has misled into believing that milk is an important source of calcium and protein. Perhaps this would be true if most milk was not altered from its original form: RAW, unheated, from chemical-free cows, and unprocessed. To make matters worse, like most other altered foods, milk is "fortified" with synthetic vitamins. In *Home Safe Home*, Debra Lynn Dadd (p.241) writes, "it is very rare to find pasteurized and homogenized milk that has not been fortified with vitamins A and D, a process that adds propylene glycol, alcohols and BHT...There is evidence...that the process of homogenizing milk, wherein a substance called xanthine oxidase is released, may contribute to heart disease in humans." Moreover, the vitamins introduced into milk are isolated chemicals, not nutrients.

Pasteurized milk, as found on most grocery store shelves contains altered fats and is robbed of its inherent, natural supply of vitamins and enzymes.

Most milk is a poor source of calcium

According to researcher Dr. Richard P. Murray, "Many authorities state that milk and milk products are the best source of calcium...However, as common to most all authorities, no consideration is given to the fact, nor ever mentioned, that heat-processed milk calcium has impaired bioavailability by reason of precipitation and catalytic enzyme loss. Analogously, a deer is the best source of venison, but not after it's run over by a truck and lies on the side of the road for two weeks. There's a difference." (Murray,1990, Part B) In other words, once milk has been processed, it no longer can be utilized by the body as a nutrient-rich food. If you must drink milk, it is ideal to have it in the raw form from a reliable source (Certified Grade A organic), and free of steroids, hormones and other chemicals that are either injected into cattle or introduced into their feed. (For a detailed discussion of how dairy and meat products are subjected to myriad chemicals which the consumer ingests, you may want to read the best-selling book *Diet for a New America*, by John Robbins).

Similarly, other dairy products are equally as altered by the time they find their way to the store shelves. Cheese and butter undergo processing that change these otherwise healthy foods into nonfoods. For people suffering the slings and arrows of outrageous indigestion and upper respiratory problems from dairy products, it is best to either avoid dairy or try raw, Certified Grade A versions to be found at good health food stores.

MEAT

Red meat has come under a lot of fire in recent years by natural and allopathic healthcare doctors alike. It has been blamed for contributing to heart disease, clogged arteries, cancer, overweight, diverticulosis and indigestion. Is this blame well-founded? Only if you consider just part of the whole picture. There are many variables involved in the health picture of meat eaters to determine the source of their illnesses. Organically grown/"free-range" beef, is a good food, devoid of those chemicals commonly fed to, or injected into, most other beef products (including hormones, antibiotics, etc.). Scientific studies blaming meat products for illnesses are often misleading, because the real concern is not the meat itself, but rather what is done TO it, how its biochemical composition is altered, and how it crowds other important (especially fiber-containing) foods out of the diet. Although the human body is often taxed by the consumption of too much meat, which is a chore to digest, assimilate and eliminate, these problems are often secondary to greater health concerns—toxic substances that are in meat products before they even reach the shelves of the grocery store.

Researcher David Steinman writes (p.4):

> The U.S. Department of Agriculture (USDA) is responsible for the safety of the nation's meat supply. Yet its history is replete with incidences of allowing the food supply to be dangerously contaminated with bacteria as well as carcinogenic animal drugs, growth stimulants and hormones…So poorly has the USDA monitored the safety of the nation's meat supply that in October 1993 a new labeling law went into effect requiring meat packers to warn consumers of the bacterial contamination of their products. An extensive review of governmental reports on the antibiotic and sulfa

drug residues in meat allowed to be sold to the public indicates that edible portions can be contaminated by an array of drugs, including penicillin, streptomycin, tetracycline, neomycin, oxytetracycline, gentamycin, sulfamethazine, sulfathiazole, and sulfaquinoxaline. Other unsafe drugs used regularly in livestock include dimetridazole, ipronidazole, and carbadox, each of which is carcinogenic and may leave residues in edible portions. Bite into a piece of nonorganic beef today and you are getting a taste of the rancher's modern pharmacy.

Meat eaters today are not eating the quality product of yesteryear—from cattle that grazed peacefully in wide open spaces under the big Montana sky in 1899. Today's cattle are treated inhumanely and are raised on feed that is full of chemicals, pesticides, synthetic fertilizers, animal byproducts and even fecal matter.

Author Debra Lynn Dadd writes,

Although some animals are fed soybeans, corn, barley and other grains, others may be fed ground cardboard, old newspapers, sawdust, and recycled animal wastes. Researchers are even studying human sewage for ways to process it into animal feed...Commercial feed may contain growth-stimulating hormones, coloring agents, fungicides and pesticides, drugs and medicines to treat diseases and flavoring agents to make it more appealing to the animals....In all, more than 1,000 drugs and another 1,000 chemicals are approved by the FDA for use in feed. And many of these substances wind up in our bodies via burgers, chicken dinners and bacon breakfasts...The General Accounting Office of the U.S. government has identified 143 drugs and pesticides that are likely to leave residues in raw meat and poultry. Of these, 42 are known to cause or are suspected of causing cancer, 20 can cause birth defects and 6 can cause mutations.

Anyone treating his household pet in the same manner as today's cattle would surely invite the Society for the Prevention of Cruelty to Animals and the Humane Society to his door along with the local news media hungry for a big bust! Today's cattle are raised indiscriminately for profit; and the bigger, leaner and cheaper they can be raised goes to feed the bottom line, not the health of the consumer (or the cow).

Author David Steinman writes, "Men whose bodies are built on testosterone end up dosing themselves with estrogen; women also end up ingesting estrogen, which causes breast cancer—thanks to the beef industry's use of hormonal implants for fattening up non organically raised beef. Some of the other drugs…cause cancer at other sites in the human body; all represent consumer health hazards."

Preparation

Even good, healthy meat can be transformed into a poor food, depending on how it is cooked. Research shows that broiling and barbecuing (over gas or coals) meat may produce a cancer-causing substance called *benzo(a)pyrene*. Good fats on meat are easily turned into bad fats once cooked at high heat, potentially leading to an imbalance of essential fats involved in nerve transmission, hormonal function, the health of the skin and balance of cholesterol levels. In its natural state, meat can be a good food, yet once altered by the beef industry and the cook, it can readily become a nonfood. For the ultimate nutrition, Native Americans and other indigenous, ancient cultures traditionally ate meat in its fresh, raw form—from muscle to brain, and from liver to glands. Slow cooking, stewing, baking and roasting is preferable (health-wise) to barbecuing or broiling.

SUGAR

As with so many foods, it is important to distinguish between good sugars and bad sugars. Natural, raw sugar is a food; refined sugar is a nonfood (most biochemists would simply call it a chemical). Most sugar consumed in the American diet is refined/processed and may be a contributing factor in a whole array of illnesses including diabetes, tooth cavities, skin problems, attention deficit disorder, anxiety, hypoglycemia, hyperactivity, nervousness, lightheadedness, chronic dropping blood sugar, insomnia, overweight, fatigue, poor appetite, increased appetite, adrenal fatigue, PMS, chronic fatigue, chronic wounds/sores and more. Even worse than refined sugar are those inventions of modern science called "artificial sweeteners." These may cause cancer, headaches, flu-like symptoms and other horrific side effects. As bad as refined sugar is, it is still better than artificial sweeteners!

Dr. Richard P. Murray, wrote in *Roots Newsletter*:

> It has been written: "No commodity on the face of the earth has been wrested from the soil or the seas, from the skies or from the bowels of the earth with such misery and human blood as sugar."
>
> The "Slave Trade" of 20 million Africans was in most part—at least two-thirds—for providing workers for the sugar cane fields of the West Indies and the sugar planta-tions of Louisiana. For 300 years, following the consent of King Ferdinand of Spain in 1510, ruthless trafficking in human lives across the sea maintained the labor pool that plowed the fields for the growing production of sweet, white gold.
>
> Just 15 years ago, the world consumed more than 92 million metric tons of sugar. Americans, on the average, consume more than 77 pounds of refined sugar per year from the sugar bowl. Another 45 pounds per year is con-

sumed by the American by way of corn sugar sweeteners added to supermarket (processed) foods and drinks. That totals, per person, 5 ounces per day or about 8 tablespoons every 24 hours.

Biochemist Roger J. Williams, Ph.D., University of Texas, wrote: "It is…interesting and distressing for those who are concerned with food as a world problem to realize that we Americans have exported to other countries one of our most serious nutritional habits—excess sugar consumption. Greater sugar consumption spells poorer nutrition, because sugar provides calories that have been stripped of all the minerals, amino acids and vitamins."

He says, as most everyone knows, "Sugar promotes tooth decay as it affects adversely both the external and internal environment of the teeth."

Williams also cites research data which implicates excess sugar consumption with atherosclerosis and heart attacks. Quoting Yudkin and co-workers in England, he tells us: "It would mean, for example, that a person taking more than 110 grams of sugar a day (4 oz.) was perhaps five or more times likely to develop myocardial infarction (heart attack) as one taking less than 60 grams a day."

Average Americans use about 140 grams of sugar per day.

Fifty years ago, Dr. Royal Lee had some thoughts about sugar: "Starches are better than sugars as energy foods because they are assimilated slower and do not overload the pancreatic function of supplying insulin. Glucose is the quickest to diffuse through the intestinal wall; levulose the slowest. Because of its rapid absorption rate, glucose is the only sugar that definitely causes diabetes; at least in test animals. Glucose is the cheapest sugar, and therefore it is used as a filler or adulterant in foods. Dried fruits are often saturated with glucose to increase their weight."

McLeod's Physiology tells us that four ounces of glucose are found in the bloodstream fifteen minutes after we eat it. The same amount of levulose requires four hours. Levulose (4 ounces) has the same sweetening power as 7 ounces of cane sugar, while 4 ounces of glucose (sweet taste-wise) would be equivalent to about 1 ounce of cane sugar.

"Soft drinks are an insidious source of glucose requiring much more glucose than cane sugar or sucrose."

Harold Lee Snow, M.D.,...from his testing, summarized:

1. refined sugar is a drug, not a food;
2. obviously is responsible for many diseases of infancy and childhood;
3. sugar, like alcohol, is habit-forming;
4. refined sugar causes vitamin and mineral deficiencies;
5. results in tooth decay, diabetes, indigestion, flatulence, skin diseases, anemia, obesity, respiratory membrane weakness, arthritis, tuberculosis, cancer, high blood pressure, fatigue; and
6. refined sugar is difficult to avoid because it is found in all packaged, canned and processed foods.

When you eat refined sugar, a host of vital nutrients are pulled out of the cells then enter the bloodstream, including magnesium, potassium, calcium, phosphorus and more. As a compensation, the body releases adrenaline. It is easy to see how eating refined sugars can make children hyperactive with all of that adrenaline coursing through their bodies. You can also see how the cycle of eating sugars can eventually wear down the adrenal glands and deplete the body's supply of many essential vitamins and minerals. In the least, the result is adrenal, or chronic, fatigue.

Sugar is hidden in most commercial foods...

People on the lookout for bad sugar quickly recognize white sugar, but sugar processors are clever enough to disguise refined sugar by calling it other names in their products. Beware that refined sugars also go by the names of sucrose, corn syrup, fructose, maltose, powdered sugar, glaze, glucose, dextrose, lactose, sorbitol, xylitol, mannitol, caramel, dextrin, polydextrose, invert sugar, high fructose corn syrup, brown sugar, and even often "sugar in the raw." Any kind of sugar can be refined, not just cane sugar.

It is common to forget that most of the sugar consumed may not even come from the sugar bowl. Even if you are not *adding* sugar to your foods, you can bet that food manufacturers are doing the job for you. Refined sugars are to be found in the ingredients of most grocery store packaged foods, including ketchup, barbecue sauce, cookies, cakes, breads, cereals, soda, bagels, bread mixes, pasta sauces, rolls, beverages, snack foods, so-called "natural" carbonated beverages, steak sauces, gravy mixes, salad dressings, pudding, "energy bars," diet powder drinks, jams and jellies. It is not uncommon for soft drinks to contain 8 teaspoons of sugar in one 8 ounce can, and your ketchup may contain a teaspoon of refined sugar per tablespoon of ketchup!

The sugar alternative? Try Sucanat, stevia, raw fruits, or raw honey. Not only are these real foods sweet, but they also contain important vitamins, minerals and other nutrients; and these forms of sugar contain natural factors to properly utilize themselves (i.e., they do not burden the body as do refined sugars).

Desserts

Sweet, sugary desserts such as cookies, candy and cakes serve absolutely no nutritional purpose. If you must have sweets, try at least to eat a healthy alternative to the typical desserts laden with chemicals, refined sugars, bad oils and food coloring. If you CRAVE sweets, then consider the fact that your body may be deficient in one or more nutrients. For instance, many people with vitamin B deficiencies and adrenal gland disorders crave sweets because they are tired all of the time and rely on artificial stimulation. And, of course, women often crave chocolate and other sweets around their menstrual periods (as a result of hormonal fluctuations, mineral deficiencies and/or adrenal fatigue). But instead of considering sugar as a "quick fix," consider the right kind of diet along with whole food supplementation (see Appendix for supplement companies) to rebalance your body's biochemistry and thereby eliminate the dependence on refined sugar.

HYPERACTIVITY, PROCESSED FOOD & MEDICAL EDUCATION

If you have children or grandchildren in school, here's something to think about: Teachers spend more time with our children than we do during the waking hours. This is may be a frightening prospect, if you are not fortunate enough to have good teachers leading your child delicately down the path of learning and discriminatory thinking. Having had children in school—both private and public schools—I know first-hand that too many teachers frequently thwart every effort we make toward reversing the horrible eating patterns and foul-nutrition we perpetuate in this country. Children are rewarded with candy and other sweets by bringing in cupcakes, cakes and cookies for nearly every holiday celebration and birthday party. Many children are used to sell sweets in the form of cookies and candy as major methods of fund-raising. Our children are taught falsehoods which special interest groups endeavor to pass on from generation to generation to fatten their pocketbooks—that nonfoods are harmless *real* foods that should be associated with fun times and special occasions.

When the meat and dairy industry position their products as a major food group (for the purposes of increasing sales) by infiltrating the school system with their "nutrition" literature, teachers help perpetuate their propaganda by offering it as "fact" to our children. It is no secret that teaching "aids" including flyers, posters and coloring books are often supplied by the Dairy Council, McDonald's, the American Heart Association and other self-serving institutions. The result is that we have children and their parents convinced that pasteurized milk and cheese, hamburgers, ketchup, French fries, margarine and ice cream milk shakes are acceptable nutrition, which they are not. The fact that so many school-related nutrition policies and literature are endorsed by dietitians is equally disturbing, given the fact that certain dietitian associations are supported with funds by entities (including the poultry, beef, fast-food, margarine and sugar industries) which produce some of the most notoriously offensive non-foods known to human beings. This relationship amounts to no less than allowing the wolves to watch over the sheep.

Too many teachers fill our kids with more sugars than their little bodies can handle. Then it comes as a surprise that there is an "epidemic" of moody, attention deficit disordered, hyperactive children and children coming down with the flu like clockwork every fall and winter. Combine this scenario with what is fed in the school cafeteria, candy bars stuffed in lockers, candy vending machines, cookies packed in lunch boxes, classrooms and playgrounds bombed with poisonous pesticides, fluoridated and chlorinated water and stressful peer pressure, it is a wonder at all that our children make it out of the "war zone" in good health.

If you are a teacher, please do your homework—learn from objective sources about nutrition, sugar, dairy, processed wheat, beef and the effects of foods and nonfoods on the body's biochemistry. As a teacher, you are charged with forming the backbone of our next generation—both figuratively and literally.

We need to consider the source of our educational materials. Find out who funds the research that comes up with "proof" that one substance or another is good or bad for us. There are countless manufacturers in our country who go around looking to commission some laboratory, university or scientist to prove that their product is good for the consumer. If they are successful in buying this research, then they can be successful in selling their products. Medical and scientific institutions are paid great amounts of money (grants) to substantiate the goodness or effectiveness of their products so that you and I will believe it is not only fit for consumption, but also beneficial to our health. Case in point: In April, 1998, the Welch's company (makers of grape juices and jams), paid a university to "discover" and report to the media that their grape juice was beneficial for the health of the human heart. What's more amazing than the process of the study is that the national news media broadcasted the voice of the doctor giving testimony to these wonderful findings as scientifically substantiated news!

NO NEWS IS REAL NEWS

Many television programs tout themselves as "investigative" news shows, and are renowned for running lengthy segments on the benefits of certain new wonder drugs. These programs amount to no less than infomercials for drug companies and surgical techniques. Meanwhile, the viewer mistakenly regards them as unbiased news. It makes one wonder whether such programs would ever be aired if it weren't for the millions of dollars poured into commercial advertising on the same networks that broadcast the reported benefits of their products. The next time you watch television, be aware of the difference between real news and "reports" carefully disguised as real news. You just can't afford to believe most of what you see and hear on the evening news or major television networks, magazines or newspapers pertaining to the benefits of drugs, medical treatments, artificial foods, genetic engineering, irradiation, a new "medical breakthrough" or medical procedures. Chances are that the "news" is not really news, but misleading or manipulative propaganda and promotion. We get what we pay for.

Read the labels

The difference between foods and nonfoods becomes apparent once you get the idea that real foods don't really need labels. It's either real food or it's not. Raw fruits, vegetables, nuts, grains and seeds do not need labels for you to know that they are natural unless they are packaged by a food manufacturer. (This term, by the way, always strikes me funny—the truth is that only nature "manufactures" food, not companies.) Once a food is altered, added to, "enhanced," enriched with so-called vitamins, cooked, processed, refined, dyed or molecularly changed, then it becomes a nonfood. Nonfoods are not nutritious, they are unhealthy. Read the labels on all foods you buy. If there are names of chemicals that are unfamiliar to you, then don't buy them. Foods shouldn't contain chemicals.

Be on the lookout for these nonfoods as well:

Some of the nonfoods we commonly find on the shelves of our food stores include preservatives, colorings, dyes, artificial flavorings, salts, tenderizers, aluminum, refined sugar (including high fructose corn syrup, corn syrup, white sugar, turbinado, glucose, brown sugar, etc.), refined oils, processed flour, wax, synthetic fertilizers, pesticides, hydrogenated and partially hydrogenated oils, growth hormones, synthetic and fractionated vitamins, coal tar, fillers and chemicals not listed, but hidden within the ingredients. Because unknown chemical substances may be in products even if not listed on the label, it is best to shop at a healthfood store and purchase products from manufacturers with a history of commitment to (and specializing in) pure and natural foods.

When you consume nonfoods, you are putting a demand on your eliminative organs which are saddled with the burden of throwing off these substances. If your diet is heavily laden with additives, you can believe that your systems of elimination—your lungs, bowels, kidneys, skin and lymph system—are overburdened already.

Pesticides, used ubiquitously on all kinds of produce, fruits, nuts, and vegetables,—and found in non-organic meats—kill more than just "pests." They also kill beneficial microorganisms, pollute the environment and contribute to more health problems than we have yet identified. In *The Wellness Advocate* (1994), Dr. Judith A. DeCava wrote: "Pesticides can cause cancer, damage the liver, adversely affect the nervous system, injure the lungs, compromise the immune system, lead to gastrointestinal diseases, kidney damage and much, much more. The toxic substances are often stored in fatty tissues of the body, which may be metabolized as fuel or other functions of the body, and thus the poisons may be released. Fat-soluble pesticides may be stored in individual cells where they can interfere with vital operations including oxidation and energy production. Any tissue, any function of the body, may be touched."

Foods that commonly make people sick (often without them knowing it)

If you are chronically sick, consider the following substances that may be in your diet and eliminate them for at least three months to test the results:
- Coffee (especially non-organic)
- Alcohol
- Refined flours
- BHT, BTH
- Hydrogenated (and partially-hydrogenated) oils, including most peanut butter, imitation butter, margarine, salad dressings, mayonnaise, "spreads," snack foods and fried foods
- Iceberg lettuce (high in pesticide residues) even when rinsed & virtually devoid of nutrient value
- Refined sugars
- Diet sodas
- Artificial sweeteners
- Pork

- MSG (monosodium gluconate, commonly found in Chinese restaurant foods, barbecued potato chips, bullion cubes and yellow rice)
- Most canned soups (may contain MSG or aluminum). Look for healthfood store brands.
- Roasted nuts (frequently contain rancid, indigestible or altered oils)
- Fried foods: heated oils are commonly indigestible and can disturb many bodily functions which rely on good fats for function (such as the hormonal and nervous systems)
- Tap water
- Chlorine
- Fluoride (often in toothpaste, drinking water and mouthwash)
- Tobacco
- Children's fruit-flavored drinks (often contain dyes, refined sugar and other artificial ingredients)
- Soft drinks

Nutritionist Dr. Bernard Jensen once wrote: "Whatever goes in your mouth should be nutritious. If it is not, you are cheating yourself."

FATS AREN'T NECESSARILY BAD:
SOME ARE ESSENTIAL TO HEALTH
(& THE TRUTH ABOUT CHOLESTEROL)

The subject of fat in the diet is one of the most misunderstood topics in the field of nutrition, perhaps because this subject is very complex and not easily stated. Refined food manufacturers, clinics and diet book publishers have capitalized on the public's ignorance and confusion about fats by raking in fortunes selling the erroneous notion that all fats and cholesterol are bad and they should be banned from the diet and replaced by low-fat and artificial fat substitutes. There is prevailing confusion on this issue because food manufacturers, diet gurus and many healthcare practitioners fail to make the critical distinction between fats that are detrimental to the health versus those that are VITAL, or essential to health and life. While some fats are indeed bad, such as margarine and hydrogenated oils, others are absolutely necessary to provide the building blocks of life, such as essential fatty acids.

OMEGA FATTY ACIDS

Biochemically speaking, fatty acids are the precursors (building blocks) for fats and oils. "Essential fatty acids" is a term used to describe precursors of "good" fats necessary, or essential, for human health, and in particular, cellular and physiological function. In layman's terms: We must have certain kinds of fats so that our cells will work.

According to *Anthony's Textbook of Anatomy and Physiology* (p.42), "An essential fatty acid is one that the body cannot synthesize [make on its own] and that is essential for survival. One's diet, therefore, must include essential fatty acids."

While the world is going crazy over marketing claims about the evils of fats, our population is suffering from a lack of essential fatty acids in our diets.

John Finnegan, author of *The Facts About Fats*, writes:

> Studies have found that the main nutrient most of us are deficient in is the Omega-3 fatty acid. An inadequate intake of this nutrient has been established as a main cause of most modern diseases. Today, because of food processing, the average diet contains only one-sixth the amount needed and one-sixth the amount the average diet contained in 1820. (And in many diets, one-twentieth to one-hundredth the amount needed.)....There are only two main sources of Omega-3 fats: cold water fish oils and organic flax seed oil. Flax seed oil is the richer source of Omega-3 fats: it requires less processing, tastes better, contains no toxic substances…, is more stable and is less expensive..

The Omega-6 fatty acids are also of critical importance in maintaining good health. Most modern diets contain ample (if not excessive) amounts of Omega-6 fatty acids, but insufficient amounts of Omega-3s. Omega-6s must be taken with an adequate amount of Omega-3s or they can have a deleterious [negative] effect on health. An acceptable ratio amount researchers [have determined] is about four to six parts Omega-6 to one part Omega-3 in the diet. Although some historical diets point to a one-to-one ratio.

With today's typical diet, however, this ratio is so out of balance that the body cannot survive in good health. What's worse is that, due to the means of oil processing, most oils sold to the public (even including most of those in the healthfood store) are not health-promoting! If you are shopping for oil, look for unrefined, organically grown brands. Cold-processed oils are not unrefined. Other than extra virgin olive oil, which is unrefined, the label should state "unrefined."

Omega-9 fatty acids are found in olive, hazelnut, sesame and almond oils and have been recognized to benefit liver and gallbladder functions as well as provide energy and prevent heart disease.

NOT ENOUGH OF THE RIGHT FATS

John Finnegan writes, "Of all the foods that we consume, none is as severely processed and converted into poisonous substances as are the fats and oils. Use of high temperatures and chemical solvents, as well as exposure to light and oxygen in the processing methods of nearly all oils produced today, destroys much of the Omega-3 and -6 essential fatty acids, and creates rancidity, poisonous trans-fatty acids and many other toxic compounds."

While the world goes mad on the no-fat/low-fat craze, informed researchers are telling us that we don't get enough of the right fat in our diets. In *Understanding Fats & Oils*, Michael T. Murray, N.D., writes:

> Many experts estimate that approximately 80 percent of the American population consumes an insufficient quantity of essential fatty acids. This dietary insufficiency presents a serious health threat to Americans. In addition to providing the body with energy, the essential fatty acids—linoleic and linolenic acid—function in our bodies as components of nerve cells, cellular membranes, and hormone-like substances known as *prostaglandins*. Prostaglandins and the essential fatty acids play an important role in keeping the body in good working order, such as

- producing steroids and synthesizing hormones
- regulating pressure in the eye, joints or blood vessels
- regulating response to pain, inflammation, and swelling
- mediating immune response
- regulating bodily secretions and their viscosity
- dilating or constricting blood vessels
- regulating collateral circulation
- directing endocrine hormones to their target cells
- regulating smooth muscle and autonomic reflexes
- being primary constituents of cellular membranes
- regulating the rate at which cells divide (mitosis)
- maintaining the fluidity and rigidity of cellular membranes
- regulating in-flow and out-flux of substances in and out of cells
- transporting oxygen from red blood cells to the tissues
- maintaining proper kidney function and fluid balance
- keeping saturated fats mobile in the blood stream
- preventing blood cells from clumping together
- mediating the release of pro-inflammatory substances from cells
- regulating nerve transmission
- stimulating steroid production
- being the primary energy source for the heart muscle

As well as playing a critical role in normal physiology, essential fatty acids are shown to be therapeutic and protect against heart disease, cancer…multiple sclerosis and rheumatoid arthritis, many skin diseases and others.

It becomes rather obvious that the problem (not just with overweight people) is that the wrong kinds of fats are being consumed while at the same time, the right kinds of fat are not. This poor pattern of eating, which is so commonplace, leads to deficiencies of essential fatty acids. Fat is a natural, necessary and essential component of food, along with carbohydrates and proteins. Without the consumption of essential fatty acids, we could not live. The lack of essential fats in the diet leads to countless malfunctions causing or contributing to a long list of ailments, including (but not limited to) psoriasis, dermatitis, acne, PMS, eczema, sinus conditions, headaches, behavioral disorders, multiple sclerosis, arthritis, heart disease, liver disease, gallbladder disease, hypertension, impotence, vascular (blood vessel) disease, arteriosclerosis, vision problems and neurological disorders.

Dr. Michael Murray writes, "Early in the twentieth century, Americans consumed about 125 grams of fat a day. Today, the consumption is closer to 175 grams, a 40 percent increase, or about 50 extra pounds a year. Proportionally our ingestion of saturated fats has remained relatively stable. Our ingestion of unrefined polyunsaturated oils rich in the disease-preventing essential fatty acids has decreased dramatically. Conversely, our ingestion of refined, adulterated polyunsaturated oil products has risen sharply, correlating with the dramatic rise in many degenerative conditions including cancer, heart disease and stroke. These refined and processed compounds actually inhibit the body's ability to use the essential fatty acids that are consumed." Altered oils fail to meet our nutritional needs at the cellular level, and even worse, they are regarded as toxic substances by our bodies.

AVOIDING FAT FOR WEIGHT CONTROL

Our nation is obsessed with weight loss programs inducing people (predominantly women) to avoid ALL fats, from butter to nuts. In a recent issue of *Townsend Letter for Doctors*, author/nutritionist John Finnegan wrote, "The frightening news is that for the past three generations (since the advent of refined oils), the vast majority of the population in North America has not been given adequate nourishment for complete brain development. The part of the brain that Omega-3 [fat] affects is the learning ability, anxiety/depression, and auditory and visual perception."

Pregnant and nursing mothers who are in fear of gaining weight are, more often than not, avoiding the types of fats essential for their own health and the development of their babies. A Mayo Clinic study suggested that Omega-3 fats should be supplemented in every pregnancy and that refined and hydrogenated fats be avoided for at least this critical period. (Even better advice would be to forever avoid these particular bad fats).

BUTTER VS. MARGARINE & HYDROGENATED OILS

Processed food manufacturers, diet book authors, weight loss clinics/ programs and many dietitians, have created a debate over whether butter is healthier than margarine. Margarine is a man-made product that many biochemical researchers believe is one of the most dangerous inventions of food manufacturers, as it threatens the health of many physiological functions and cellular structures, including the arteries and nervous system. Author John Finnegan wrote that "Butter is a good wholesome food that mankind has been eating for thousands of years without adverse consequences. But now, people eat margarine—a lifeless poison, packed with carcinogens [cancer-causing agents], fit only for lubricating the front wheel bearings of your car."

Author Rudolph Ballentine, M.D., explains that by "bubbling hydrogen through vegetable oil," a 'new fat' is created...[A] recent elaborate statistical analysis of the incidence of heart disease and the consumption of hydrogenated fats in England has shown a dramatic and detailed correlation between the two....It is interesting to note that in the Southeastern [United] states, the region where margarine consumption is highest in relation to population and to butter consumption, there is an area where the incidence of heart attacks is so high that it has been termed 'an enigma.' It seems increasingly likely that eating margarine, instead of preventing heart attacks, actually accelerates the process which causes them."

Scientists employed by food manufacturers have discovered that when hydrogen is added to vegetable oils, they become solid at room temperature and do not spoil as quickly; but the bad news is that hydrogenated (or partially hydrogenated) oils are unhealthy substances which disrupt the biochemistry. John Finnegan explains, in the process of hydrogenating oils "natural oils are heated under pressure for six to eight hours at 248-410 degrees F and reacted with hydrogen gas, using a metal-like nickel or copper as a catalyst. If this process is brought to completion, as in vegetable shortening, you have a partially hardened oil, as in most margarines."

Trans fatty acids (fatty acids that have been altered molecularly during hydrogenation), writes Finnegan, "compete for enzymes, produce biologically nonfunctional derivatives and interfere with the work of the essential fatty acids in the body. Because of our association of the word 'polyunsaturates' with health, we are misled into thinking that we are buying a health-giving product of good quality, a product that is actually health-destroying...There are so many possibilities of different compounds that can be made during partial hydrogenation that they stagger the imagination. Scientists have barely scratched the surface in studying all the changes induced in fats and oils by hydrogenation. Needless to say, the industry is hesitant to fund thorough and systematic studies on the kinds of chemicals produced and their effects on health. The industry is equally hesitant to publicize the information which already exists on the topic."

Biochemical researchers such as Dr. Richard P. Murray have long claimed that hydrogenated oils, such as those found in margarine and other altered fat products, contribute to the destruction of the cells lining the walls of blood vessels. Once these blood vessels crack, tear and ulcerate, the body may attempt to "patch"(repair) them with cholesterol and calcium. Instead of blaming the problem on bad fats in the diets, doctors usually lay the blame on high cholesterol. It's a case of "killing the messenger."

WHAT MAKES A FAT BAD?

It seems that most of our health problems stem from a DEPARTURE FROM NATURE. Once we stop eating truly natural, whole and pure foods, we create all sorts of nutritional disruptions. Oils (fats) that are created in nature are usually destroyed, altered or removed from food during processing. Since most people eat processed foods, most people are also lacking essential fats in their diets.

In refining (processing) wheat, for instance, food manufacturers remove the part of the wheat plant that contains essential oils (fats). Their reasoning is for the sake of practicality and economics. Oils spoiling on the grocery store shelf are bad for profits. Therefore, they are removed from the wheat during processing, yielding a product that has been one of the scourges of modern health—refined wheat. As humans, we NEED the oils as much as we need vitamins, minerals or any other life-sustaining nutrient.

Good fats come from natural, whole, pure foods—the kinds nature provides without human intervention and alteration. Bad fats come from frying, roasting nuts, hydrogenation, partial hydrogenation and products such as margarine, fake butter, non-stick sprays, barbecued fats, rancid oils, etc. Good fats come from real butter and milk (preferably raw, certified grade A), unprocessed (unrefined) oils such as extra virgin olive oil, raw nuts and nut butters, seeds, fish and good supplements of unrefined flax seed oil, borage oil, and wheat germ oil.

Like most things in life, there are "two sides to every coin." While everybody is on the fat-free frenzy, it is important to realize that there are essential fats that your body just cannot do without. If you're avoiding butter because some margarine company has convinced you that it is bad, then you have become the effect of their marketing nonsense. It seems rather obvious, but we tend to forget, that food manufacturers are biased in their claims. Their goal is to sell you their products; and they've discovered that the little phrases "no fat" or "low fat" are very attractive to people who have no knowledge of the truth about fats—some fats are good and some are bad.

The moral of the story is NOT to eliminate the good fats by wrongfully assuming that all fats are bad. Modern, processed, refined foods are not regarded by your body as nutrition. Modern scientists have deceived us into believing that nature can be improved upon without altering the course of human health. This deception seems to be the root of most of our nation's skyrocketing health problems.

THE CHOLESTEROL SCARE

Cholesterol is a natural, vital and essential substance that is as much a part of keeping you alive as your own heartbeat. So why the bad rap? Cholesterol had not become a topic of great concern until just within the past 45 years or so. Now more than ever, the topic of cholesterol leads to a Pandora's box of deliberate falsehoods and misinformation. Although we hear too much about how cholesterol and fat causes heart disease, obesity, diabetes, arteriosclerosis and strokes, we really ought to separate fact from fantasy to save our sanity. The only thing we can say for sure about high cholesterol is that it is a profitable "illness" to treat.

THE ROLES OF CHOLESTEROL

From the research of Judith A. DeCava, Ph.D. (*Cholesterol Facts & Fantasies*), we learn that cholesterol is a crystalline substance consisting of fats and is found naturally in the brain, nerves, liver, blood and bile of both humans and vertebrate animals.

Cholesterol, which is produced mainly in the liver, is a necessary part of every human cell and is imperative in almost every aspect of metabolism. Cholesterol serves as a conductor of nerve impulses. Cholesterol helps form membranes for billions of cells where it regulates the exchange of nutrients and waste products. Without cholesterol, digestion would be a most difficult task, as it is an essential part of bile salts that break down food and fats.

DeCava writes, "Without food fats, vitamins A, D, E, F and K (fat soluble vitamins) could not be absorbed....Cholesterol is an important component of hormones produced by the adrenal glands, sex glands and pituitary gland. It is needed by the skin to convert sunlight into vitamin D and provide a barrier in the skin to prevent water and other fluids from inappropriately entering the body."

Further, writes DeCava, "…cholesterol plays a part in calcium metabolism and bone structure, in heart muscle contraction and liver function. Cholesterol deficiency leads to fatigue, obesity, nervous and emotional disturbances, digestive difficulties, impotency or inability to conceive and/or complete a pregnancy, menstrual syndromes and masculine traits in women, effeminate traits in men, blood pressure irregularities, fluid imbalances, nutritional deficits and imbalances and more."

STUDIES SHOW THAT FATS IN FOODS MAY NOT INCREASE CHOLESTEROL

Despite all of the vital and invaluable attributes of cholesterol, this wondrous substance has been repeatedly blamed for heart disease and stroke to the point of paranoia. However, research has shown that often there is LITTLE OR NO REDUCTION of cholesterol levels in the blood regardless of a change in dietary intake.

According to Dr. DeCava, "The medical establishment says to eat only 300mg or less of cholesterol in foods, yet the body produces four to seven times that amount itself. Cholesterol is needed by the body." Studies show that the more cholesterol consumed in food the less the body produces. If little or no cholesterol is consumed, the body tries to produce even more. Therefore, the body manufactures and keeps within itself a constant, regulated supply of cholesterol naturally.

HIGH CHOLESTEROL LEVELS?

Blood cholesterol levels may be affected by genetics, underactive thyroid, mental stress and work-related tasks. Cholesterol can be increased by nicotine, pain, fear, pregnancy, lack of exercise, a number of drugs, and/or alcohol. Also, kidney disease, diabetes, hepatitis, and gallbladder obstructions raise cholesterol. And levels of cholesterol commonly increase with age. Cholesterol levels have even been known to change with the seasons.

Unfortunately, most of what has been reported about the effects of cholesterol is from animal studies, BUT animals do not process cholesterol like humans. Huge amounts of dietary cholesterol only raise blood cholesterol in humans a few milligrams, while in rabbits it may be raised many hundreds of milligrams.

What is considered HIGH cholesterol? According to Dr. DeCava, until 1988 cholesterol levels up to 330 were considered normal. As of late, however, the National Cholesterol Education Program has set the "safe" level of cholesterol at an ARBITRARY 200mg/dl, combining both HDL and LDL levels with no proof or evidence for choosing that number. This new interpretation states that a reading above 200 indicates potential for developing heart disease. Further, it states that a level of 200-239 is borderline, and those over 249 are at high risk. Yet, this new medical interpretation is seen by many biochemical researchers, doctors and clinical nutritionists as ERRONEOUS, MISLEADING and FALSE.

DEBUNKING CHOLESTEROL FALLACIES

Beatrice Hunter, Food Editor of *Consumers' Research*, states, "Unquestionably, among all of the food component/health relationships, the fat/cholesterol issue has been the foremost in generating misinformation, confusion, and hoopla. Conclusions of scientific studies have been couched in qualifying phrases such as 'no conclusive evidence,' 'no definite cause-and-effect relationship,' 'uncertainties exist,' 'this finding has yet to be confirmed,' etc. Despite these phrases, tentative findings have become distorted and made to appear as firm facts, and recommendations have been made for dietary and lifestyle changes before a firm scientific base has been established."

Ms. Hunter writes, "The conventional slogans are that fat and cholesterol are bad [and] the less fat and cholesterol one eats, the better for one's health. By cutting down on fat and cholesterol, one lowers the risks of heart disease and cancer. Don't you believe it!

"The public has been badly misinformed about the role of fats. Many articles and much advertising characterize all fats as bad…what is ignored is that some fats are essential for health and provide nutrients and palatability to foods."

Ms. Hunter, quoting nutritionist George V. Mann, M.D., Vanderbilt University, writes: "saturated fat and cholesterol in the diet are not the cause of coronary heart disease. That [falsehood] is the greatest scientific deception of this century, perhaps of any century."

FRAMINGHAM STUDY IS IGNORED

In 1948, Framingham, Massachusetts, a magnificent study started with nearly 30,000 adults to determine the relationships between fats, cholesterol and heart disease. After monitoring their subjects for a number of years, in 1970, the Framingham researchers reported: "There is, in short, no suggestion of any relation between diet and the subsequent development of CHD (coronary heart disease) in the study group." Despite this admission, a vast program was already being developed, and the public was being urged to lower cholesterol levels.

By the early 1980s, both the National Heart, Lung and Blood Institute and the American Heart Association concluded that, despite the lack of definite proof, there was sufficient suggestive evidence linking diet with CHD to launch a nationwide campaign to change American eating habits.

ANTI-FAT IS BIG BUSINESS!
REAL HEALTH RISKS OR ULTERIOR MOTIVES?

The question begs to be answered: Why would so many medically-related institutions rally behind a cholesterol scare? Many health practitioners speculate that the anti-cholesterol stance supports a multi-billion dollar medical-food-drug industry. By lowering the acceptable levels of cholesterol, more drugs can be sold to lower cholesterol and more lucrative treatment programs can be put into effect—this is financially rewarding to doctors, pharmaceutical manufacturers (drug companies), drug stores, laboratories, universities, food manufacturers and hospitals. Plus, herein lies an enormous financial opportunity for processed food manufacturers who keep hammering away at the American public with advertising for cholesterol-free and fat-free food stuffs. This advertising has been so successful that the lie has become the Truth—ad agencies have brainwashed the American public into believing that all fats are bad and that fat-free products are good, wholesome foods, despite the fact that they are often filled with unhealthy ingredients ranging from artificial sweeteners to refined flour and from hydrogenated fats to artificial preservatives.

The American public has been trained to equate the word "fat" with the word "bad," while processed food manufacturers have raked in fortunes at the expense of America's health.

Beatrice Trum Hunter reports, "It is time for Americans to challenge both the official dietary recommendations as well as the advertising claims about various components of food. A healthy skepticism is needed, in order to avoid being misled. At stake is not only one's pocketbook, but also one's health."

THE PROBLEM IS WITH SYNTHETIC FATS, NOT NATURAL FATS

When synthetic or altered fats are fed to animals and people, they CAN cause cholesterol problems. Natural foods containing cholesterol also contain vitamins, antioxidants, minerals, enzymes and other factors that protect the body from toxic oxidation (and help process cholesterol). Unnatural fats destroy blood vessels.

Many researchers remind us that the French diet, full of fats, butters, creams, marbleized meats and sauces, does not create heart disease or high cholesterol; and the French maintain the lowest CHD (coronary heart disease) in any Western industrialized nation. In France the death rate from CHD is 95 out of 100,000 men. In the US it is 256 out of 100,000 men.

THE BODY CANNOT USE OR METABOLIZE altered or synthetic fats in the same way that it can handle natural fats. BLOOD CHOLES-TEROL levels fluctuate frequently in response to the body's ever-changing needs.

AVOID ALTERED FATS

The antidote to the cholesterol scare is to eat only unaltered fats and other whole, natural and pure foods because there is no scientific evidence to suggest that any natural fat (or any other REAL, unprocessed and unaltered food) causes an abnormal increase in cholesterol or heart disease. Cholesterol levels can and do increase to deal with stress, including the insults of unnatural fats and/or refined sugars, which appear in most of today's processed foods.

As long as we have scientists on the payroll of large food manufacturing corporations, we will see the invention of new forms of "foods" and food additives. Foods cannot be human-made and natural foods cannot be enhanced or enriched without tampering with human health.

THE POLITICS OF
NATURAL HEALTHCARE

All doctors and healthcare practitioners should understand nutrition in order to treat their patients. Although this sounds like a logical statement, the truth is that most doctors know very little about nutrition. Although more and more medical doctors are embracing nutrition as a means of understanding disease etiology (causation), there is a great stumbling block to progress. Because there is no big money in the practice of nutrition, pharmaceutical companies (drug manufacturers), hospitals, medical associations, dietetic associations and even vitamin and supplement manufacturers are launching extensive, deceptive public relations and advertising campaigns seemingly supportive of natural healthcare. In reality, they run contrary to the principles of Natural Healthcare. Now many healthcare practitioners are (perhaps often unintentionally) blurring the line between natural and unnatural forms of healthcare by administering or recommending the use of nonfood substances in treatment programs. If a substance—despite whether it is a drug or an herb or a vitamin—is used to stimulate or suppress a specific bodily function instead of to feed the cells, then such a substance is being used as a *pharmacological* (drug-like) agent. This is analogous to pushing (as opposed to repairing) a disabled automobile to its destination. Natural healthcare is not natural if it incorporates substances which only push or suppress the body's natural functions.

A COUNTRY AT WAR

There is currently a war of sorts between natural healthcare proponents and the established modern medical industry. Behind this war is an age-old theme—greed. The casualties are citizens who are being bombarded with misinformation, one-sided information and the propaganda that nature is unnatural and that drugs should be preferred solutions to eradicate symptoms of disease.

Most medical doctors, based on my personal experience, are intelligent people interested in helping their patients. However, except for a minority of free-thinking, independent-minded physicians, most do not think in terms of what is natural, nor are they trained to think outside of the medical paradigm to embrace nutrition and natural therapies. Doctors are not being taught (in medical school, in medical literature and journals, or in continuing education seminars) the most fundamental of all principles— that the body is a biochemical entity requiring FOOD particles to feed cells—the basic units forming muscles, bones, nerves, organs, blood vessels and so on. As such, too many doctors accept the dogma they are taught rather than trusting in their inherent logic which says natural solutions are always preferable to unnatural attempts to force the body to behave in a specific manner. These doctors commonly advise their patients that eating better foods is not a serious healthcare practice in the face of illness. Like programmed robots, they advocate the use of some drug, whether by pre-scription or over-the-counter, to address nearly every illness and symptom. Doctors who act this way are not only following the "party line" of the pharmaceutical companies, medical association and big business, but they are also misled by their own egos to think that they are qualified to give advice about nutrition—a field in which they are only novices at best.

If your doctor tells you that nutrition has nothing to do with your health, then he/she obviously is speaking out of ignorance. Instead of being intimidated by any health professional, be bold enough to ask what he/she knows about nutrition and its role in biochemistry, human physiology, symptomatology and disease causation. When a drug is offered to you, ask about its side effects. Your health depends on your sense of self-responsibility, personal research and consideration of your options.

When considering natural healthcare alternatives to their primary physician's advice, oddly enough, patients often return to their original doctor for his approval and opinion. In effect, the original doctor is put on the spot. What is he to say?—that he is wrong and some alternative therapy would be better than his own advice? If he does this, he is made to look foolish or uninformed. The original doctor is likely to condemn and criticize any course of treatment except his own. William Campbell Douglass, M.D., in *Second Opinion Newsletter* (Vol.VIII, No.6, 1998), writes: "In 98 percent of cases, the family will take the literature describing the [alternative] treatment to their doctor. He will, because of ignorance or greed, tell them the treatment is quackery, dangerous, a waste of money, experimental, etc., etc., none of which is true." Get a second (and third and fourth) opinion from an outside, objective source, not your own original doctor.

In defense of medical doctors, it is true that there are good and bad physicians, just as there are good and bad lawyers or good and bad building contractors. There are a great number of medical doctors who are open-minded and willing to work with nutritionists, natural healthcare doctors and other practitioners for the good of the patient. These are the types of practitioners who are worth knowing and working with for your health. In truth, any kind of professional advice is only as good as its source. You must consider the character, integrity, sincerity, attitude, expertise, knowledge and compassion of a doctor even more than the initials after his/her name or expertise or medical school.

PERPETUATING HATE, CONFUSION & DEFAMATION

Medical textbooks on biology, biochemistry and physiology used in modern medical schools recognize the value of specific nutrients in the role of human health. However, this invaluable information is overshadowed and supplanted by the economic interests of pharmaceutical companies, hospitals, medical associations, "charitable" foundations and other special interest groups whose wealth and longevity hang precariously on public opinion and doctors' decisions.

These special interest groups support and finance "studies" at leading hospitals and universities to prove the viability of **their** products, regulate the information taught in medical schools and perpetuate the American lie (to both doctors and patients) that disease should be treated with drugs and that all of this talk about nutrition and nature is nonsense. (For further substantiation, the reader is referred to the book *Inventing the Aids Virus*, by Peter Duesberg, 1996). Natural healthcare doctors and nutritionists (and even medical doctors who refuse to ignore the value of nutrition in human health) are publicly referred to as "dangerous quacks." This sort of defamation is both overt and covert. By keeping medical doctors from becoming involved in truly natural healthcare, pharmaceutical corporations and medical associations are preserving and ensuring their stronghold over modern medicine to maintain their ever-rising profits through drug sales and surgeries. Huge profits and exclusivity just cannot be garnered through the sale of real foods instead of patented drugs. Nutritional advice and dietary adjustments are inexpensive; while on the other hand, open heart surgery and blood thinning drugs are big money makers.

Author of *Confessions of a Medical Heretic,* Robert Mendelsohn, M.D., (p. 38) confers when he writes:

> If you look at almost any other system of medicine besides the Western, you'll find a heavy reliance on food. The "food" of Modern Medicine, however, is the drug. The American doctor, aside from a very fragmentary and usually incorrect approach to certain "therapeutic diets" (gout, diabetic, low salt, gallbladder, weight reduction, low cholesterol), completely disregards nutrition. Those who are concerned with nutrition are labeled faddists,

freaks, extremists, radicals and quacks. Occasionally, they're (more correctly) referred to as *heretics*.

THE TAIL WAGS THE DOG...

The actions of greedy power interests in this country include:

- Defaming practitioners who are not MDs, including chiropractic physicians, naturopathic physicians, nutritionists, hypnotherapists and "alternative" practitioners;
- Launching campaigns to promote the dangers of vitamins and other supplements while downplaying the side effects, deaths and disabilities caused by drugs, surgeries, vaccinations and injections;
- "Teaching" the public about the dangers of "quacks;"
- Frightening the elderly and parents of small children into receiving medical treatments for potential "medical threats" such as viruses, bacteria and contagious disease (even when the causes of such disease are admittedly unknown and treatments are based only on theory);
- Proclaiming that supplements such as vitamins and herbs are so dangerous that only medical doctors should be allowed by law to "prescribe" them;
- Destroying the reputation and work of medical doctors who dare to refuse to follow the "party line" of drug usage and surgery in lieu of natural alternatives;
- Influencing government agencies to bully non medical doctors as well as medical doctors practicing alternative healthcare. Government agencies such as the FDA (Food and Drug Administration), DEA (Drug Enforcement Agency) and FTC (Federal Trade Commission) have been used to carry out arrests and seizures against doctors (especially medical doctors) who practice natural healthcare. Somehow these agencies have forgotten that it is the American public that pays their salaries and that they are supposed to work on behalf of the American public rather than special interest groups;

- Creating icons out of medical doctors and proclaiming that they are the only professionals smart enough and trained enough to engage in any form of healthcare;
- Instilling in the public's mind that hospitals are holy places of knowledge, human respect, dignified healthcare and "state-of-the-art" institutions that work for the public good and protect the public from the evils of natural healthcare. Walk into any hospital and pick up its brochures. Notice how these self-glorifying terms are used to portray their services: "state-of-the-art, ultra-modern, leading technology, leading physicians, certified physicians, dedicated staff, trained doctors, specialized physicians, board certified, experienced doctors, ultra-modern facilities, caring environment," etc. Those of us who have read the "insider" newsletters published by hospitals and medical centers "for physicians and medical staff only" will readily tell you that these institutions are interested foremost in profits; the patient is secondary. Hospital administrators (who are not doctors in most cases, but rather businessmen and women), are in their positions to make money, not to care for people, contrary to their advertisements and public relations materials. To make more money, they open up special departments to treat specific diseases, like cardiac units, arthritis programs, fertility units, pain centers and diabetes programs. If any of these programs or departments are not lucrative, they are discontinued as fast as they were erected and the medical doctors in charge are history;
- Instilling in the public's mind that the only viable healthcare choice is that of modern medicine, using medical doctors, hospitals, nurses, and drugs. All else is, at best, referred to as "experimental" and "risky," when the truth is that statistics prove that modern medicine is itself a VERY risky alternative;
- Using terms to defame and dissuade interest in natural healthcare, such as "unproven," "dangerous," "unregulated," "voodoo," "untested," "unscientific," etc.;

- Putting medical doctors on a lofty pedestal as the final arbiter to judge the merits of all healthcare devices by using terms in advertising such as "ask your doctor," "recommended by doctors," "doctor-approved," "the brands doctors use;"
- Telling the public that only medical doctors are qualified to practice healthcare of any sort, despite the fact that physicians are not taught to understand the role of nutrition in human health nor do they generally have clinical experience in the practice of nutrition;
- Misleading the public to believe that drugs are a logical solution to disease. Even though most diseases are caused by nutritional deficiencies, biochemical imbalances and/or chronic poisoning, these problems are addressed with drugs and not those specific nutrients which are known by nutritional experts to bring the body back into healthful balance.
- Hiding, inventing and falsifying research results to befit the financial goals of medical associations, drug companies, utility and nuclear power companies, vaccine inventors, etc. (Beware that even the "natural" healthcare industry is not immune to such public deception with claims that are based solely on anecdotal stories and not proven conclusions).

CONTROLLING THE MEDIA & PUBLIC OPINION EQUATES TO HUGE PROFITS & LOYAL FOLLOWERS

Read any major magazine or tune into the major television networks, and you will notice that these media are literally controlled by pharmaceutical corporations, chemical companies, energy conglomerates and refined foods manufacturers. Without their advertising money and financial ties, the media would suffer a severe financial death-blow. Knowing this, so-called "news" shows with big-name celebrity broadcasters are used to "expose" the risks of taking unprescribed supplements and herbs, and seeking alternative healthcare practitioners. These news shows' so-called "investigative" segments hailing the wonders of modern drugs and medical procedures are no more than infomercials for pharmaceutical companies and special interest groups in the guise of public safety and information. Is it any wonder that good information about natural healthcare is rarely brought to you via your very own television set? The suppression of news and the expression of slanted views is the real "epidemic disease" in the free world. For an eye-opening exposé on this subject, the reader is invited to pick up a copy of *20 Years of Censored News* by Carl Jensen, Ph.D. (Seven Stories Press, New York). The author reminds us of Thomas Jefferson's insight when he said in 1799, "The man who never looks into a newspaper is better informed than he who reads them, inasmuch as he who knows nothing is nearer to truth than he whose mind is filled with falsehoods and errors."

When leafing through your favorite magazine, notice that on the reverse side of advertisements for drugs (medications) is a list of side effects that are staggering. After reading these side effects, ask yourself whether modern medicine sounds like a safer alternative to the prevention school of thought that incorporates lifestyle changes, stress reduction and nutritional responsibility. The next time you are watching television, pay attention to the ads for both over-the-counter and prescription drugs and be aware of how much the TV viewer is inundated with messages about the "wonders" of pharmaceuticals. Advertising for drugs is escalating every year, attempting to sway more and more people from successive generations to the modern medical model of better health through drugs. This is the irony—drugs do not provide health at all, yet the advertising messages would have you believe otherwise.

Lisa Belkin, in her article "Primetime Pushers," *Mother Jones*, relates:

> Wherever you flip on the TV dial nowadays you will find commercials for medications that you cannot actually buy. Not without the permission of your doctor…These are serious drugs, with potentially dangerous consequences, but the mood of the ads is upbeat and cheery. Cholesterol busters battle for market share. Antidepressants come with handy checklists of symptoms. Joan Lunden hawks Claritin. Newman from "Seinfeld" pitches an influenza

drug. Pfizer spokesman Bob Dole promotes cures for erectile dysfunction.

…Television ads for prescription drugs, which were all but outlawed as recently as four years ago, are now taking over your TV set. To wit: Pharmaceutical companies spent an estimated $1.7 billion in TV advertising in 2000, 50 percent more than what they spent in 1999, more than double the 1998 amount. In 1991, only one brand of prescription medication was marketed on network television…

The rush to the airwaves was triggered by the U.S. Food and Drug Administration, which, until four years ago, had required that manufacturers include nearly all of the consumer warning label in any pitch—something possible in a magazine advertisement, but prohibitive in a 30-second television spot.

By the way, it is entirely legal for drug companies to specifically name both the product and the disease in the same advertisement. BUT it is not legal to name a non-drug along with the disease it may be used with. It is not legal, for instance, for an herb company to state that laetrile is effective in cancer treatment.

WHAT MAKES US SICK: A NUTRITIONAL DEFICIENCY OR A DRUG DEFICIENCY?

If a nutritional deficiency causing a disease is not addressed with nutrients coming from real, whole and natural foods, then even with modern medical intervention using drugs and surgery, the same disease frequently reappears, or the patient soon afterward presents similar symptoms in another part of the body. Despite highly trained cardiac surgeons and multi million dollar, state-of-the-art cardiac units in hospitals, many cardiac patients are known to have multiple heart attacks even under the watchful eyes of their cardiologists; they are on their medications "for life." Despite the fact that powerful drugs are used for migraine headaches, these headaches recur over and over again. Despite the fact that a patient is put on thyroid medication, the thyroid never gets better and the patient is told that the drug is to be faithfully taken "for life." Likewise, despite drug intervention, heart arrhythmias, asthma, arthritis, diabetes, multiple sclerosis, and hundreds of other diseases are merely (if at all) controlled, but are **not cured**. The reason is that **drugs are not living biochemicals required for human health**.

Drugs and surgical operations (tactfully referred to as "procedures") are big business, and the more ignorant you are of natural healthcare and what you can do to help yourself, the happier will be those who can control the modern medical system. **No one gets sick due to a drug deficiency!**

How important is it for us to be barraged by drug commercials on TV? Very important for the drug companies who rake in billions of dollars a year, and feel the effects of their advertising in their pocketbooks. Writer Lisa Belkin, in her article "Primetime Pushers," *Mother Jones*, writes:

> Some of the most dramatic cause-and-effect can be seen in the category of allergy drugs. Claritin maker Schering-Plough launched the televised assault against sneezing in 1998 when it spent $185 million on advertising and saw sales more than double to $2.1 billion. Following the leader, Pfizer spent $57 million to promote its drug Zyrtec in 1999 and saw a 32 percent increase in sales; that same year, Aventis spent $43 million to promote Allegra, and sales increased by 50 percent.

Although the numbers of allergy sufferers have not increased to keep pace with this new drug demand, Belkin writes,

> According to Scott-Levin, a pharmaceutical consulting company in Pennsylvania, doctor visits by patients complaining of allergy symptoms were relatively stable between 1990 and 1998, at a rate of 13 to 14 million per year. In

1999, there were 18 million allergy visits. The cause of the spike, critics point out, is clearly the advertising.

The purpose of allergy ads in particular and pharmaceutical ads in general "is to drive patients into doctors' offices and ask for drugs by brand name," says [Larry D.] Sasich [a pharmacist with Public Citizen's Health Research Group in Washington, DC]...And once they are in that office, patients often get what they want. "Physicians are more interested in pleasing their patients than you might think..."

Why not please the patient? Isn't it all about making money anyway? Who cares if the patient really needs the drugs, or even worse, whether the side effects are harmful?

Investigator Dr. Carl Jensen (*20 Years of Censored News*) discovered that more than 20 years ago, "according to the Food and Drug Administration (FDA), up to 500,000 different non-prescription remedies generate at least $3.51 billion in sales every year [today this estimate is nearly $17 billion), and, according to its investigating experts who amassed 14,000 volumes of evidence on these over-the-counter (OTC) drugs, the people who purchase them are 'the victims of a gigantic medical hoax.'"

Dr. Jensen continues,

The conclusions of intensive independent studies first launched in 1972 by more than 100 leading medical researchers, physicians and pharmacologists recruited by the FDA are that 'at least half the drugs are worthless or of dubious value, and some may be harmful. Most of the products are labeled with misleading claims, and many are advertised with bold lies.' While the industry invests in massive advertising campaigns, it spends comparatively little in developing and testing new drugs: "Major OTC producers spend at least $400 million in network television spots each year...telling consumers, about fifty times a day, that medically ineffective products will really work."

Dr. Jensen reminds us that "In the magazine industry alone, drug marketers spent $163 million in 1990; by the end of 1995, that total had ballooned to $502 million, according to the Publishers Information Bureau (*Inside Media*, 2/7/96)."

Factual information today is very difficult to ascertain; while untruthful information is fed to the public and doctors alike to the point where real, objective and valuable healthcare succumbs to the weight of economic and political factors. Steven D. Findlay, an analyst and director of research and policy at the National Institute for Health Care Management tells (Belkin, p. 33) us that drug ads tend to teach consumers how to describe their symptoms so they can get medication through their doctors. He says, "'The purpose of advertising is not to inform people…It never has been and it never will be. The purpose of advertising, as we all know, is to make people buy more product so the company can make more money. It makes you desire that new product, just like that new car or that new gizmo.'" People, including doctors and government officials, lose their sense of objectivity in the face of profits.

What's being lost here in the advertising glitz is the real, cold fact that drugs are being promoted as answers to our ailments. The other side of the story is not being presented—the natural side. Worse yet, while the drug and medical institutions are running wild with their marketing and ad campaigns, they play unfairly, forcing the government to disallow equal types of advertisements for natural products. Further, drug and medical institutions carry so much weight, spending so many dollars on advertising that they FREQUENTLY force the media into running public relations stories on them to tout their "miracle cures" and wondrous benefits. The public remains in the dark because they're not being shown the entire picture—objective reporting on the pros and cons of drugs as well as the viable alternatives.

SIMPLE ADVICE IN A NUTSHELL

Here's the simplest advice in the quest for your personal healthcare: Don't believe what you see on television because the information you receive, whether advertisements, infomercials, news "specials" or nightly news, is undeniably slanted toward the use of pharmaceuticals and modern medicine. If pharmaceuticals (drugs) could actually cure disease, then, with our arsenal of thousands of wonder drugs, we would already be disease free. Yes, it's repetitious, but the point is that drugs don't cure diseases because diseases are not caused by drug deficiencies.

Support the healthcare practitioner who supports you with dietary/ nutritional advice based on real, whole foods and substantiated facts, whether it's a medical doctor, naturopath, Oriental medical doctor, nutritionist, dietitian or chiropractic physician. Doctors who are sincerely interested in your health are open-minded and not afraid to share in your success by working with other qualified professionals who may be more informed than they are. Don't let your doctor abuse you, talk down to you or make you feel uncomfortable about asking questions or challenging his/her suggestions. After all, in what other field would the customer (you) be expected to bow in subservience to a paid consultant (the doctor)?

NATURE TAKES
HER TIME IN HEALING & DISEASE

Throughout history, the ages of human civilization have been labeled according to preoccupation—the Golden Age, Dark Ages, Age of Enlightenment, Industrial Age, Nuclear Age, Space Age, Age of Information, etc. Now we have entered into the **Age of Convenience**. As a busy, highly stressed, over-worked, malnourished, foul-nourished, industrialized society, people not only lean toward convenient solutions to their problems, but are very open and receptive to "solutions" based mainly on convenience. This fact has allowed us to become manipulated by corporations; and has caused us to settle for unreliable, albeit attractive, and short-term solutions to our problems. We have fallen prey to the quick-fix mentality—we want results, and we want them NOW!! To appease this mentality, scientists and innovators have invented a great many quick-fix institutions, fast food restaurants, packaged and processed foods, drive-in banks, speed-reading programs, fast crop turn-over farming technology, prescription pharmaceuticals and over-the-counter drugs offering quick relief, instant financing, one-day surgery suites, outpatient care, and the infamous quickie market. With careful comparison, you'll see a single thread of commonality running through them all—they all cater to, foster and encourage our inherent sense of impatience.

The Age of Convenience is giving way to the Age of the Great Decline, as the quick-fix mentality trains and deludes us into believing that fast is preferable to right; and that out of sight/out of mind is a logical and intelligent stance to take against our problems. This attitude gives us an easy means of turning our backs on—and separating ourselves from—nature and the natural process. Yet, as natural, biological beings, we cannot afford to take such a stance without contributing to our early demise: fast food, quick-fix medical solutions and impatience lead to disease and a slow, painful death (of ourselves and our civilization).

BACK TO NATURE

Getting back to nature, we need to accept the fact that real healing takes time. There is no way around this issue. Although modern medical pundits tell us that a shot at the doctor's office will clear up an infection, and that we MUST schedule our surgery "right away," we in the natural healing arts feel that quick-fix solutions and emergency operations are in no way a resolve. Drugs, medications and other synthetic "solutions" to illness manifest in some other disease at some other point in time. Surgeries do not cure diseases at all. If modern, Westernized medicine cured disease, then, with all of the drugs now on the market, we would all be happy, healthy and carefree. But the truth is that drugs only work to help us live with our diseases and discomforts, not to eradicate them. The reason for this is very clear and bears repeating: No one gets sick due to a drug deficiency!

AREN'T THEY MISSING THE POINT?

There's a popular television commercial for a new over-the-counter indigestion pill in which a yuppie daughter shows her mother how effectively a particular antacid works. The mother's response is, "Wonderful, now I can eat pizza again!" This is typical of the way people are trained to think. In essence, they are proclaiming, "Now that I have the antidote, I can poison myself whenever I want," or, "Now that I can't feel the pain from the fracture in my leg, I can go jump out of another tree." This mind set reflects a complete ignorance and careless disregard for disease and healing, with an emphasis only on alleviating symptoms in which natural biochemical processes within our bodies are circumvented (bypassed).

In fact, even the "successful" outcomes of research studies on so-called "natural" supplements are sold to the public with the same frame-of-mind: When we are told that a supplement or a drug "works," we are only being fed part of the whole story. We are told, for instance, that chondroitin "works" for arthritis sufferers, or that co-Q10 works for heart patients. But what do they mean by the term "works"? If they mean that a supplement or drug gets rid of a symptom, then they claim success in scientific trials and successfully sell the product to the public. Yet, real healing DOES NOT mean only that the symptom has disappeared. Rather, the most important part of the equation is whether the CAUSE of the illness has been addressed and whether the cells have been **nourished** to the point where they have repaired damaged tissue; AND whether the patient has ceased contributing to his/her own self-destruction by means of poor diet, injury, toxic exposure, etc.

Each year, in medical centers nationwide, modern surgeons perform thousands of cardiac bypass operations and angioplasties to alleviate the symptoms of collapsed, occluded (blocked) and diseased arteries. Some of these surgeries are life-saving (although some doctors would even debate such a statement), and the skilled surgeon should be applauded for his contribution and technique. However, the question longs to be posed: Where was the surgeon ten or twenty years ago when the patient was shoveling pancakes, hamburgers, bacon, margarine, steaks, fries, soda pop and cakes into his mouth? Or is it the surgeon's fault at all? Perhaps its the fault of all of the big corporate, medical and government interests that keep us from the truth—that eating and nutrition are the link to building and preserving health.

If care is taken in preventing heart disease, cancer, lung disease, diabetes, tooth decay, arthritis and any other number of chronic ailments, nature provides a kind of health and vitality that no man-devised means of correction can even approach in its effectiveness and permanence.

Neither disease or good health "happens" in an instant. Nature takes her time. This is the natural state of being of which we are all a part. You've no doubt heard the old poem that proclaims only God can make a tree? Well, if you believe this, then maybe you will entertain the notion that even God doesn't perform that feat overnight. A seed is nurtured by air, water, light and nutrients in the soil. Then it sprouts and continues to develop into a tree. There must be some sort of wisdom in this transcendent, gradual-but-steady process of growth and healing. Drugs may "work" fast, but wisdom tells us that it is impossible to force the course of nature to speed up a real cure at the cellular level, engaging the cells to reproduce, grow, repair and provide immunity.

The human body, with all of its cells, tissues, organs, vibrations, nerves, energy systems and other elements, is as much a part of nature as a clump of clay, a weed, a flower, a tree, a mountain, the air, the sun and the ocean. The only problem is that we tend to forget this, as our egos delude us into think-ing that we are not a part of nature and that its laws somehow do not apply to us. To illustrate this point, study the faces of flood or tornado victims and you'll notice that they are full of surprise at nature's awesome effect on their homes, land and possessions—they are out of touch with the course of nature and do not consider man's relationship with it. They believe that, just because they build a house and conduct business in a given location, nature should stop its course. You would have thought this lesson would have been permanently ingrained when the ancient, thriving city of Pompeii situated dangerously near the rumbling Mount Vesuvius, was buried in a mere few hours in volcanic ash. Nature knows no human limits.

People complain to their doctors that they don't feel so well after con-suming a lifetime diet of nutritionless brands of coffee, soda, potato chips, cereal, milk, spaghetti and meatballs; and they complain to their lawyers that they got food poisoning at their favorite seafood restaurant when they shouldn't have been eating there in the first place; and they drag their feverish children into the ear doctor after giving them swimming lessons in chlorinated water then feeding them cookies, milk, soda pop, bagels, cupcakes, birthday cakes, candy bars and processed foods served in plastic and aluminum containers. Are you seeing the pattern here? We take plenty of time to build our ill health, but we want to be cured immediately, if not sooner. When someone walks into my office suffering with some chronic illness and I tell him that to get better it may take six months to a year, he may balk and say, "That long?" My response is, "How long do you think it took for you to make yourself sick?" There's a lot of undoing and rebuilding to be done. Too many people are so far removed from nature that they expect foods and whole food concentrate supplements to work like drugs or they don't want to go through with the program. They are out of touch with the course and design of nature.

The lesson here is: We are all part of nature whether we want to believe it or not.

7 RULES FOR HEALTHY EATING

An entire book could be written on rules for eating, but this short and simple chapter provides the basics. Here's how to avoid the effect of bad eating habits…

RULE #1
EAT FOR HEALTH

When you eat, consciously consider what your food is doing for your body, not just for your sense of taste. Too many of us regret having devoured a delectable malted milk shake only to wake up the next morning with painful sinus congestion; or having eaten a rich, sumptuous five-course meal only to experience more gas than the Hindenburg blimp. How many fathers across the nation perform the after-meal ritual of unbuttoning their bursting trousers and slumping into gastric despair? Except perhaps in childbirth or to save another human being, pain is rarely worth the experience in hindsight. Try to think ahead before you choose to eat something bad for you. Before sinking your teeth into a pie, for example, consider that its refined sugar creates an acid condition in the body and robs your cells of minerals, feeds unfriendly bacteria in the bowel, becomes stored in the fat cells, contributes to blood sugar imbalances and decays teeth.

RULE #2
EAT MOSTLY RAW FOODS

Raw, fresh and organic fruits, vegetables, seeds and nuts, and certified Grade A organic raw dairy products provide the most nutrient value in the diet. When foods are cooked, heated, watered down and exposed to air, we destroy enzymes, essential fatty acids and oils, vitamins and other vital nutrients. When foods are processed, they are converted into non-foods that offer very little health value and a lot of health-destroying potential. Raw foods offer your digestive tract the fibrous constitution necessary to keep the walls of your bowels unobstructed and they contain vitamins, good fats and amino acids not found in processed foods such as crackers, cookies, French fries, pancakes and soda. By eating at least 50 percent of your foods in the raw, natural, whole state, you will increase your energy, avoid most weight problems and give your body food for building and rebuilding tissues.

RULE #3
AVOID DEVITALIZING YOUR FOOD

Foods that are overcooked, processed, microwaved, fried and in any other way altered from their natural state create a host of digestive problems ranging from gas to constipation and from intestinal cramps to bloating. Devitalized foods lead to cellular starvation and disease.

RULE #4
EAT WHOLE, NATURAL FOODS

Our bodies, being the natural temples that they are, thrive on natural, whole foods. And nowadays, due to the widespread proliferation of toxic synthetic fertilizers and pesticides in our soils, we must also look to the organic farmer as a viable source of wholesome nutrition. Eating chemicals, pesticides, fungicides, dyes, taste-enhancers, MSG, drugs, preservatives, hormones and sprays creates a toxic load that your body has difficulty processing and eliminating. These toxins back up in your channels of elimination, find their way into your cells (bone, fat, brain, liver, etc.) and plant the seeds for disease. Nature's foods (grown organically) provide what your body needs; human-made and human-enhanced foods are no longer natural. Nature is already perfect in her bounty; altering her delicate balance builds the foundation for disease. The best foods to eat are ones that do not come with a list of ingredients, and are found in their natural, whole form without additives or alteration.

RULE #5
EAT A VARIETY OF FOODS

The body requires a variety of foods for a variety of minerals, vitamins, enzymes, fats, proteins, trace elements, amino acids and other nutrients that cannot be gleaned from one food source alone. If you are looking for carotenes, try dandelion greens and Swiss chard, for example, in addition to carrots. Or try fresh pineapple juice, guava or bell peppers in addition to fresh orange juice for your vitamin C. Each food contains its own particular quality and quantity of nutrients. But beware that when news reports and books extol the virtues of specific foods for their nutrient contents, these nutrients are found in the unaltered food, not the processed varieties found in the typical grocery store. For instance, orange juice may be full of wonderful nutrients, yet pasteurized (cooked by heating) orange juice is no longer the same food.

Peter Ways, M.D. (Bliss, 133) writes, "No simple food or group contains all the nutrients you need." A variety of foods ensures that your body receives balanced nutritional input.

RULE #6
CHOOSE REAL FOODS THAT ARE BEST FOR YOU

We are all individuals and therefore have individual nutritional needs. It is best to avoid adopting a generalized eating regimen or even a disciplined diet just because some "expert" says it is "what most people need." A diet of 80 percent vegetables may be good for some people, but not for everyone. A vegetarian diet may be ideal for some, yet your body may require animal products. Although we have been oversold on the importance of protein foods by the meat and dairy industries, the need for protein is an individual one. Since most meats are cooked and overcooked, they add very little to the overall health picture and worse, are the source of altered fats and digestive difficulties. Worse yet, most animal products are tainted with drugs, pesticide residues and other toxic substances. This means that in many cases it's not the meat that's so bad, but rather all of the poisons associated with the meat. If you require meat, be sure to buy "free-range," organic varieties. An array of vegetables may be adequate to provide you with an abundance of protein building blocks (amino acids), chlorophyll, fiber, enzymes, minerals and vitamins (all referred to as phytochemicals) and may be all that you need for the sustenance of life. On the other hand, you may find it necessary to supplement the vegetables with fruits, nuts, seeds and meat (poultry, fish, beef, etc.). In any case, the only sound nutritional advice that applies to everyone is to eat real, unprocessed foods to supply yourself with nutrients.

Many people frown upon meat-eaters as immoral and barbaric. The truth is, however, that anytime we eat—and whatever we eat—we must consider that, as part of the food chain, we must consume other live beings (either animals or plants), and this is one of life's necessary sacrifices. Plants have feelings too. Many people pray before they eat (although comedian Rodney Dangerfield tells us that his mother was such a bad cook, in his house they used to pray *after* they ate), and this is usually to thank the Creator for their food. But if you want to contemplate on this, you may consider thanking the food itself for giving its life so that you can sustain your own.

RULE #7
DRINK GOOD WATER & PLENTY OF IT

Good water is as rare to find today as good air, good soil and good tax exemptions. We are finding more pollutants in our drinking water today than ever before due to inadequate standards of quality control and toxic residues that have contaminated water supplies from here to the North Pole. If you drink water out of the tap, please realize that you cannot rely upon your government or water company to provide you with water that is fit for human consumption.

In *Food Fundamentals*, (54) Judith DeCava writes, "A comprehensive survey by the Center for Responsive Law, as reported in January 1988, detected some 2,100 chemical compounds in U.S. drinking water. Of these, 190 are known or suspected to be dangerous, the rest have not been adequately studied for health risk."

What makes drinking water so unhealthy? Consider the fact that every time it rains, pollutants from factories, automobiles, power plants, lawn mowers, pesticides, fertilizers, airplanes and other contaminators are washed down to earth and fall into our waterways. Each time we flush the toilet we add to the dumping of tons of sewage water into our oceans, lakes and streams. Medical wastes from hospitals, cruise ship wastes, industrial waste, nuclear waste, farming chemicals and pollutants from the average American citizen, ranging from house paint to photography chemicals, are thoughtlessly dumped into our environment, adding to a toxic build-up that can't help but find its way into our drinking water.

Heavy metals, such as lead, are often found in water supplies. Copper is another major contributor to drinking water toxicity—from copper pipes, copper refrigeration coils, and copper containers.

Other contaminants making people sick include aluminum, fluoride and chlorine. According to DeCava, (1994, 55), "Chlorine is used by municipal water treatment facilities to eliminate bacterial contamination…Chlorine can provide the agent for producing alloxan in the body that inactivates zinc and destroys the replicative integrity of the insulin-producing Beta cells of the pancreas, leading to diabetes. Chlorine is referred to as the 'basic cause of atherosclerosis, and resulting heart attack (as well as) stroke…Evidence strongly suggests that chlorine creates the compound hypochlorite, which in turn creates free radicals that not only oxidize essential fatty acids, but also creates dangerous toxins in the body…"

E Environmental Magazine (March/April 2001, pp. 12-13) reports, "There's no question about it, bottled water has become a hot commodity. Americans pay $4 billion a year for the privilege of drinking it. Sales of bottled water have grown nine-fold in the past 20 years, and tripled in the last 10, making it the fastest-growing segment of the beverage industry. According to a 2000 consumer usage survey, a third of the people who buy bottled water do so because they trust that it comes from a clean source…" But, research is showing that even bottled water has come under suspicion, much of it containing pesticides, solvents, fluoride, arsenic, industrial waste and excessive amounts of microbes and nitrogen. "Chemicals typically used to disinfect water may react unpredictably with such substances, adding their own potentially dangerous element as well. Chlorination, which can create byproducts suspected to be carcinogenic, is used primarily on municipal water supplies (from which 25 percent of bottled waters are actually sourced)." Like any other commodity, when buying bottled water, it's a matter of "buyer beware."

And what of fluoride? **For a review of fluoride** in drinking water, turn to the chapter on TOXIC WASTES.

Although controversy still reigns on the drinking water issue, the best source is from reverse osmosis (RO) processing. There are easily-installed systems available for home use; or you can check into your nearest water store and buy bottles of RO water. Drinking from the tap, however, can be linked to cancer, headaches, gastrointestinal disorders, metal poisoning and a host of other illnesses.

Due to our biochemical make-up, we must consume water to remain alive. By drinking an adequate volume of water, we aid our kidneys in elimination, keep our bowels moist, allow elimination of wastes to exit our skin, replenish lost water through perspiration, avoid muscle cramping, reduce acid build-up in our bodies, keep our skin from wrinkling and cracking, avoid dehydration, balance minerals, assimilate vitamins, and wash out natural salt wastes that are natural by-products of metabolic processes.

DOCTORS MAKE A LIVING
ON FOOLISH PEOPLE
—HOW TO REVERSE A DISEASE—

Nutritionist, author, pioneer natural healthcare doctor, crusader for common sense and full-time philosopher Bernard Jensen, D.C., Ph.D., has written thousands of words (and scores of books) on nutrition and healthy lifestyle, but one of the most memorable things he ever wrote was this bell-ringing statement: "Doctors make a living on foolish people." Knowing the works of Dr. Jensen, these words are not to be taken as an insult, but rather as an insight to people's curious habit of acting without conscious thought or consideration for the effects that are sure to come. In contrast to the traditions in the Far East, Western medicine is based on treating the effect of disease—an often futile reaction to ignorance of prevention and a lack of wisdom.

WHAT HAPPENS WHEN YOU
WAKE UP & SMELL THE ROSES?
—WHEN YOU DECIDE TO "CLEAN HOUSE"…

Paying off the lasting effects of poor nutritional and lifestyle choices takes motivation, self-responsibility and honesty with yourself. Even more so, it takes persevering through the often painful or uncomfortable consequences of your actions which may be reexperienced on the road to recovery.

Have you ever heard of Hering's Law of Cure? It is a principle known to homeopathic healthcare whereby disease is said to exit the body during or after a cleansing diet and a new lifestyle of healthy eating has been initiated. During the natural course of detoxification, disease is redirected from its chronic or degenerative stage back through to the acute stage. At this latter stage, if very toxic, the patient may experience a healing crisis—karmic payment has begun. Hering's Law of Cure states (Bliss, 76):

1. Healing moves from the deepest part of the organism (the mental and emotional states as well as the vital organs) to the more superficial parts (the skin, muscles, ligaments and extremities);
2. Healing flows from the upper part of the body to the lowest parts;
3. Healing progresses in reverse chronological order of the appearance of symptoms.

To anyone who has begun a program of renewal, cleansing and reversal, all of this means, that it is possible that you will *feel* a little worse before you begin to *get* better.

Diseases often follow the course of these four main stages: acute, subacute (more recently referred to as *subclinical*), chronic and degenerative. In the acute stage, we recognize the **symptoms** of a disease as the body's attempt to rid itself of toxins or to heal itself through a natural process. (Sometimes this occurs in the form of inflammation). In the subacute (subclinical) stage, a person has attempted to "treat" his acute illness, yet by the use of drugs or other means of artificial suppression or stimulation, has driven the disease further into the tissues and has blocked nature's means of ousting it. In the chronic phase, the body is now operating with constant pain, discomfort and/or disability as the disease has been allowed to take up residence in the tissues. Often the disease spreads into (or affects) other bodily systems. Finally, in the degenerative stage, we find destruction of tissues caused by a neglect to heal the body. Degeneration, of course, leads to the breakdown of bodily systems and ultimately, death.

In all four of these stages, the body's elimination channels are burdened as they attempt to expel toxins from the bloodstream and the tissues. By the time a disease reaches the degenerative stage, the elimination channels have been so overburdened or overworked that they may even cease to function.

Hering's Law of Cure is an analogy for changing the overall health pattern from one leading down the path of destruction to one leading to optimum health. In this light, it has been referred to as the *reversal process*. Yet, keeping in mind that nature seeks balance and harmony through action, we come to realize that, to reverse disease, we must personally take the initiative and steps to work through it. This is the role that self responsibility plays in the scheme of things—although you may be guided, the ultimate truth is that no one can do it for you. A wife cannot do it for her husband and a mother cannot do it for her child. In the final analysis, it is the individual who must embrace the awareness and attitude of good health. To experience the healing (reversal) process, you must bite the proverbial bullet and face up to the pain and consequences you have irresponsibly and ignorantly created over a period time by your poor choice of eating, thinking and lifestyle. And you must realize that real healing does not come overnight; often it is a long and drawn-out struggle that takes commitment, determination, faith and appreciation of finally moving in the right direction. If you create pain, disease or disharmony—even to your own body—you must pay for it some time.

Dr. Bernard Jensen writes (1995):

> The law of destruction and degeneration is impartial where the human body is concerned…the law of cause and effect takes care of us. We start in the flu [beginning of disease with accompanying symptoms] stage and suppress it, dry it up, and eventually we advance to the subacute state if our habits of living remain unaltered. We're still living on the knowledge of our mothers. We're living according to a culture in keeping with our ethnic backgrounds. The

Germans continue with their pickled pig's feet. The Danish still enjoy their Danish pastry. The Viennese have their pastry problems too...As we observe sugar consumption in the world, we find excessive sweets in many countries. America has her problems with hot dogs, hamburgers and cola drinks, as well as the avalanche of sweets that tempt us and these are the greatest catarrhal producers we can force on the body.

...We take a suppressant when we manifest a cough, a cold, bronchial troubles, and then we advance to the flu stage. We become susceptible to the flu. We 'earned' it by breaking down the body's natural defenses. The natural means of prevention inherent in our bodies is crippled or destroyed...We have broken down the resistance in our bloodstreams. We live in a body that is no longer capable of staying well naturally. The toxic materials build up over a period of years, augmented by suppression and catarrhal-producing diets.

What comes next? Many times we go through an array of 'treatments'...Doctors make a living on foolish people.

How can Nature perform her duty in the body built from depleted foods and the way we are living and thinking in many cases? There is only one road back...a change of lifestyle. Starting on the path of a better way of life, we reverse our route in search of healing crises...the route we must pass through the healing crises...elimination process in reverse.

You have to regenerate a clean body, one that is extremely active and ready to go to work...a body that can rejuvenate and replace old tissue with new tissue.

European homeopathic physician Constantine Hering was the champion of this (Hering's) law of cure. It is a metaphor for life itself, as we so often see the relationship between how thoughts manifest into physical action. A mental or emotional distaste leads to physical avoidance. Ignorance leads to foolish action. And a thought precedes an electrical impulse which precedes physical movement. Mental stress and emotional upset can lead to physical illnesses. The mental image of eating chocolate ice cream can motivate one to actually visit an ice cream shop and partake in the dessert. The most fundamental question becomes: How much control do you have over your mind, awareness, attitude, thoughts and impulses? This is where disease actually begins to take root. From here it steadily progresses until health declines until the entire body and its systems are impacted and congested.

Dr. Ross Trattler (35) writes, "According to homeopathic philosophy it is the inner person (vital force) that is ill, so the cure must take place from within, outward. If properly treated in this manner, disease follows a set path of elimination. Homeopathic physicians believe that disease elimination proceeds from more important to less important organs, from above downward, from within outward, and in reverse order of its origin. Thus…since all chronic disease has its origin on the surface and then progresses deeper, as proper cure is effected, first the inner manifestations of disease will be removed while the external manifestations will resurface, only later being removed as final cure results. This progression of symptoms tells the doctor that the disease is in fact once and for all being removed."

With this philosophy in mind, it is not uncommon for a patient to begin a course of treatment involving diet and nutritional supplementation to feel worse before feeling better. Often the patient experiences a retracing of symptoms which were long ago experienced at the outset of the disease between the subclinical and chronic stages. If the patient becomes frightened of the newfound "symptoms" brought on by the initial stages of repair, or becomes overly uncomfortable during the reversal process, he may quit treatment and declare that the treatment was making him sick when, in fact, he is not experiencing illness, per say, but rather the initial stages of healing. By analogy, we may say that an impacted wisdom tooth is creating major problems for a dental patient. But before the problems are gone, the oral surgeon must first damage the patient's tissue by cutting the gums and working to remove the source of the problem. It is clear that the body must be disrupted in order for full healing to take place.

POWER OF THE MIND & SPIRIT

The power of the mind is not to be underestimated in the role of healthcare. The mind, directed by spirit (our true essence, or life force), is the instrument which brings about physical manifestation. Without being mindful of health, health will be a hit-and-miss proposition, because the body will be following the pattern of an unbridled mind that seeks to satisfy the senses paramount to acting responsibly.

Deepak Chopra, M.D. (1994, 4) writes, "All of creation, everything that exists in the physical world, is the result of the unmanifest transforming itself into the manifest. Everything that we behold comes from the unknown…when we realize that our true Self is one of pure potentiality, we alight with the power that manifests everything in the universe."

In harmony with the laws of nature, Hering's Law—the reversal process—is not a quick fix healing. A person who has "sinned" against (compromised, abused, etc.) his/her body cannot bring a healing to it overnight. The overnight healing concept is a fallacy fostered by modern medical practices which fails to address the cause of a disease and only serves to mask or erase the symptoms. Just because a drug makes you feel better, don't be fooled into thinking that you are actually healed, because drugs are not nutrients and therefore cannot feed the cells; they are inanimate chemicals.

It takes time to "create" a diseased body and it takes time to rebuild health—often up to a year or more. This is a very difficult concept for many a Western-cultured mind to grasp, because we have become accustomed to, and sold on, the concept of instant gratification.

By consciously and patiently enduring the healing crisis, and allowing nature to take its course, an individual experiences the dramatic connection between his/her poor eating habits and illness.

THE BEST SUPPLEMENTS ARE WHOLE FOOD CONCENTRATES
(RATHER THAN SO-CALLED VITAMINS)

What is the difference between a living organism and dead matter? What is the difference between a single chemical and a complex group of nutrients? The answers to these questions seem too obvious to deserve a response, yet in regard to the effectiveness and credibility of supplements, even among the "experts," the difference remains unclear. Before going into the details, keep this principle in mind: That which is truly natural is also whole and balanced; and that which is created in and by nature cannot be duplicated, fractionated (split apart), isolated, improved upon, enriched, fortified or rearranged without compromising its balance and integrity. All natural things are "complex," meaning that they do not exist alone, but rather as parts of interrelated groups. The inter-relationships are what makes vitamins, minerals, amino acids and other food components function as nutrients. Vitamins and groups of vitamins, in supplement form, lack their inter-related parts because they are no longer contained within their original food complexes.

Scientists have become so empowered, epitomized, financially supported and revered that their creations have somehow become recognized and sold to the general public as greater than those of nature. But the truth remains that no scientist has ever come close to creating the essence of life out of lifeless matter. Whereas inanimate objects such as automobiles, clocks and computers may be disassembled and studied to understand their intricate parts, living organisms cannot be treated in the same manner without first destroying them. A duck, for instance, cannot be taken apart, organ by organ, nerve by nerve and muscle by muscle and still retain its identity as a living and functioning being.

Keeping with this analogy, whole, natural foods and nutrients coming from live plants and animals contain biochemicals (life-giving substances) which function only because of their complex, balanced and complete composition. Once such foods are split apart to isolate and extract their vitamins, minerals or other constituents to use in pill form, these constituents cease to maintain their biochemical integrity. To make this statement even simpler, many biochemical researchers have maintained, in the face of adversity, that a vitamin cannot be called a vitamin unless it has **never been removed** from its original food complex—it must remain within its original food along with all of its other cofactors in order for it to still be regarded by the cells of our bodies as nutrients. Pioneers in the field of nutrition and herbology have maintained that if the vitamin, or mineral or other food factor has indeed been isolated/ fractionated from its original food form, then the body regards it as a drug, not a nutrient. Even if a vitamin product is labeled as "natural," *if it is not still contained within its original food complex*, then it is no longer really a vitamin, but, at best, only a fraction (isolated part) of a food that fails to meet the complete nutritional needs of the body. Certainly, it stands to reason, and it has been proven in scientific study, that synthetic substances created out of nonliving materials to resemble a vitamin will always be lifeless and incapable of supporting life. By analogy, it may be possible to construct a new automobile part such as a radiator hose in the laboratory setting, but the same process cannot be used to create a life-form, such as a food complex, containing vitamins.

According to biochemist Dr. Robert A. Ronzio (442), "Natural vitamins are those occurring in food. All substances classified as vitamins have been isolated from animal or plant sources, and most have been chemically synthesized in the lab to establish their structures....Nutritionists often recommend obtaining vitamins from foods for several reasons. Foods supply mixtures of vitamins, minerals and other materials that may have beneficial effects...Foods supply materials that are not vitamins, yet are important...There are numerous advantages in obtaining nutrients from food: It is practically impossible to get an overdose. Food supplies... substances [other than just vitamins] that may have beneficial effects and are not found in a pill or capsule."

WHO'S FOOLING THE PUBLIC?

Estimates vary as to the consumption of vitamin products in this country, from a low $216 million to a high of $5 billion per year, depending on the source. Some researchers such as Dr. Ronzio suggest that 60% of all medical professionals, including medical doctors and nurses, take supplements. *Whole Foods Magazine* reports: "Today, an estimated 46 percent of adult Americans take nutritional supplements." Yearly, Americans gulp down an astonishing $5 billion in pills and remedies from healthfood stores, according to New York market researcher, Packaged Facts, Inc. Regardless of the exact dollar figure, not only is the use of supplements ubiquitous and monetarily substantial, but the numbers climb higher every year, owing to self-medication and self-diagnosis, widespread advertising and marketing campaigns promoting supplement use, and with modern medicine and the pharmaceutical industry jumping on the vitamin bandwagon.

But what is the quality and efficacy of these so-called vitamin products? According to Dr. Richard P. Murray, biochemical researcher and physician with more than 40 years of experience in clinical nutrition, "One of the most perilous deceptions of those who place pesos above principles is the passing off on a gullible public, phony, synthetic vitamins or crystalline-pure fractions of vitamin complexes and ballyhooing that the body does

NOT KNOW THE DIFFERENCE." Vitamin-takers may not know the difference, but their cells do!

When people think of vitamins and minerals, they usually think of capsules and tablets that can be purchased in a healthfood, grocery, or drug store, or through a mail order catalog. Most of these so-called "vitamin" supplements, including A, B, C, E and so forth are NOT really vitamins, but rather fractionated or synthetic CHEMICALS which YOUR BODY DOES NOT RECOGNIZE as nutrients, even if the manufacturer calls them "natural." At the risk of being redundant here, it must be stated that whole foods contain vitamins, but vitamins NEVER contain the myriad nutrients and synergists that are present in whole foods.

WHOLE FOOD COMPLEXES CONTAIN VITAMINS AS WELL AS OTHER ESSENTIAL NUTRIENTS

A **whole food complex** is a term used to describe the fact that real, whole, raw, unaltered foods contain a vast array of nutrients which are interrelated, interdependent and synergistic. The relationships of nutrients are complex—not simply defined or identified. Some of the factors found in whole food complexes that are known to work together (synergistically) include, but are not limited to: vitamins, minerals, enzymes, amino acids, proteins, essential fatty acids, lipids, pigments, bioflavonoids, antioxidants, fiber and more.

To understand how vitamins work, consider that the body recognizes WHOLE FOOD COMPLEXES as complete units to feed your body right down to the cellular level. Whole food complexes are found in foods and in those few supplement products that are whole foods concentrated into tablet form. (Yet, the buyer must also beware that many supplement manufacturers who claim that their products are made of whole foods are also guilty of incorporating fractionated/isolated vitamins within their pills. In other words, they mix whole foods along with synthetic vitamins and minerals. Such manufacturers are advertising to the consumer that they are something they are not.)

Food, and natural, whole food supplements, include enzymes, coenzymes, antioxidants, trace mineral activators, minerals, vitamins and thousands of other nutrients and biochemicals woven together BY NATURE into a "COMPLEX." They contain essential and dynamic elements necessary for the body to obtain and use what is needed for tissue and cell repair, healing, growth, regeneration, immunity and maintenance. Plus, the COMPLEX even contains substances, properties and energies not yet identified by scientists, but recognized and required by the body when ingested. Further, according to Traditional Chinese Medicine, whole foods also contain "qualities" that make them significant to health promotion, such as the qualities of hot, cold, dampness, dryness, bitter, sweet, sour, etc. Such qualities are not nutrients, but rather very real and notable traits of nature's foods that are certainly absent in vitamin and mineral pills.

Real vitamins exist in their original "COMPLEX" form. In other words, they have not been removed from the food that they originally come from, AND they have not been created or changed in a laboratory; nor have they been altered by processing, heating, chemicalization, etc. Once a vitamin is removed from its food, it is no longer a real vitamin, but rather a FRACTION of a food. Your body does not regard such a substance as a complete vitamin any more than you recognize a steering wheel to be the same as an automobile. In order for the automobile to function, it must be whole. It cannot be taken apart or rearranged. A fraction of the automobile is not enough to drive you where you need to go. You need the whole thing put together and working in harmony in order to drive anywhere. Similarly, like a steering wheel, a fraction of a food (a so-called "vitamin") cannot be used by your body in the same way as that same vitamin when it is still INTACT in its original food complex.

Dr. Murray said on more than one occasion, "At the very best, synthetic or pure vitamin fractions can function in the human body as only a drug or pharmaceutical agent…certainly not as a physiological supporting nutrient. At worst…counterfeit supplements can seriously impair the most important of body functions by contributing to biochemical imbalance."

WHAT DOES 'NATURAL' MEAN?

The word "natural" is very misleading when it comes to supplements these days. When vitamins come from "natural" plant sources, manufacturers label their products "natural" despite the fact that they separate (remove) the vitamins from the other ESSENTIAL ingredients in the food complex from which they are derived. Synthetic and fractionated supplements are DEAD chemicals. Your body thrives on LIVE food. Unfortunately for the consumer, when it comes to nutritional supplementation, MOST supplement manufacturers fail to make the distinction between whole food complex formulas and partially natural and synthetic vitamins and minerals.

The truth is that supplements are either natural or they are not. Supplement manufacturers do a good job of confusing the issue. To be almost or partially natural is like being almost or partially alive; or almost pregnant. Few practitioners have the time and wherewithal to investigate what makes supplements valuable to human biochemistry. Instead, they rely heavily on supplement manufacturers to provide them with information, facts, figures, schedules and potency. It is the patient (end user) who suffers when the supplements they are advised to take are not whole food complexes, but rather fractionated/isolated substances or synthetic formulations.

There are very few companies who currently formulate truly natural, complex supplements from food concentrates. There are droves of others that claim their products are natural, yet they are in actuality FROM nature or foods, but no longer natural. Some companies mix fractionated vitamins and minerals in with food concentrates. And there are even companies that manufacture entirely synthetic supplements and still claim that they are "natural."

In Empty Harvest, (127) authors Bernard Jensen and Mark Anderson write: "…vitamins function as biological mechanisms only when whole and complete, combined with their synergists, as in whole food. Isolated into synthetic chemicals, they fail as catalysts. The only hope for a vitamin effect in our body from a synthetic is to recombine, once in the body, with synergistic factors that may be available."

And what about non-synthetic, so-called "natural" vitamins? Over the years, a handful of biochemical researchers and clinical nutritionists have held fast to the claim that "it isn't natural if it isn't a food complex." Regardless of whether the supplement is purely synthetic or fractionated (isolated) from a natural plant, the failure to work as a nutrient stands as the ultimate test of whether that particular supplement has the innate ability to build, repair, aid and maintain cellular activity. To use Dr. Murray's words, "the body knows the difference." Any supplement short of whole AND natural may as well be a drug, because to the body's biochemistry and physiology, this is exactly what it is.

Whole Food Nutrition: The Missing Link in Vitamin Therapy

The following excerpts have been taken from Dr. Vic Shayne's book, *Whole Food Nutrition: The Missing Link in Vitamin Therapy*, to further explain the difference between natural, so-called natural and synthetic supplements:

> Whole foods, found in their natural, undisturbed, unprocessed state, contain a host of interactive nutrients too numerous to categorize. Some of these nutrients are vitamins, others are minerals. And there's much more. Once scientists isolated vitamins, minerals, amino acids and enzymes in a laboratory, they were able to test their functions and efficacy against disease and symptomatology. Yet somewhere along the way, modern science and marketing have allowed (persuaded?) us to forget that nutrients NEVER exist in isolation in their natural states. There can be no argument that isolated and synthetic vitamins produce pharmacological effects which show promise against disease symptoms. However, for any doctor or patient seeking a truly natural approach to healthcare, we must consider the synergistic effects of nutri-

ents contained in their natural, whole states before deciding how, when and why to use supplementation. The human body and its environment is so extremely complex and dynamic, that many practitioners, including myself, would rather surrender to the innate intelligence of nature than to presume that it is even possible to achieve wholistic results with isolated, chemical supplements. (page 8)

ARE SOME VITAMINS TOXIC?

Over the past few years, many reports have been published extolling the toxicity of vitamins, with the media scaring the daylights out of an unwitting public popping vitamin supplements as a "shotgun" approach against disease and for perceived prevention and immunity. As usual, the media are telling only part of the truth. Food complexes containing vitamins are not toxic; synthetic vitamins, however, MAY be toxic in certain doses and to certain individuals. Certainly, scientists have shown that toxic side effects are possible with the over-ingestion of vitamin A, D, B3, etc. In addition, it has been proven that vitamins, minerals and amino acids, when not taken in a balanced form, may lead to biochemical imbalances and create a health-threatening chain reaction.

This is a very real possibility, given today's zeal for fad supplements, megadosing, supplement abuses, self-diagnosis, and self-prescribing. For instance, the layman who reads that niacin is an important B vitamin that everyone needs, is really getting just a part of the whole picture. Left out is the important consideration that the rest of the other B vitamins as well as their cofactors are needed. This same person may next read that tryptophan is important for synthesizing niacin; so he then runs out for tryptophan supplements. There is no end to this chase. In another scenario, an athlete may "discover" the need for zinc which he then supplements by the handful only to accidentally impair his supply of vitamin A, vitamin C, hormones, iron and copper. Copper deficiency, in turn, can increase blood cholesterol. From here, many physiological systems may be altered, interrupted or damaged, including the adrenal glands, endocrine system, prostate health, brain chemical balance, blood cells and cardiovascular system, to name only a few, as each nutrient is linked to another in an infinite and wondrous system.

In another example of creating imbalances within the body's delicate biochemical system, an overdose of vitamin E may cause bleeding as in vitamin K deficiency. Vitamin D excess (doses 2-3 times the Recommended Daily Allowance) can be toxic when it leads to high blood calcium levels and calcification of soft tissue. "Moderately high consumption [of vitamin D] over a long period of time may increase the risk of atherosclerosis." Vitamin A toxicity is a concern with synthetic forms of vitamin A, especially in pregnancy, where it may potentially lead to birth defects. Yet, vitamin A as a natural, food constituent is very important in the diet of pregnant mothers.

Manganese overdose may interfere with iron absorption. And excessive calcium intake may interfere with manganese. Large doses of potassium can lead to electrolyte imbalances, especially for those with kidney disease, diabetes or heart problems. A complete description of how isolated vitamins and minerals are dependent and interrelated is seemingly impossible to calculate due to the variables both known and unknown.

Not only do vitamins and minerals exist as parts of delicately balanced cofactors and constituents found in whole foods, but so do amino acids (the building blocks of proteins). It is common today, especially among athletes (professional and amateur), to ingest large amounts of isolated amino acids in an attempt to build and repair muscle that is damaged in the catabolism that takes place with exertion, injury, vigorous exercise and strenuous activity. Amino acid researchers Eric Braverman, M.D. and Carl Pfeiffer, M.D. caution: "Because many of the amino acids are absorbed and metabolized in a similar fashion, there is a great deal of competition between molecules. Sometimes, one amino acid can cancel the effect of others. This adds to the overall complexity of prescribing amino acids to treat disease. For example, amino acids compete for absorption with others in the same group, e.g., the aromatic amino acid group (tryptophan, tyrosine and phenylalanine) and can inhibit one another's passage into the brain."(Shayne, pages 9-10)

UNKNOWN, BENEFICIAL FOOD FACTORS

As mentioned, not only are whole, real, raw foods sources for vitamins, minerals and other known nutrients; they are also sources of unknown factors. How do we know that there are unknown factors? Because researchers have shown that nothing like real, whole foods can provide the body with what it needs for cellular health and function; and the credit for such health cannot always been defined. For instance...

In his extensive research and cultivation of cereal grasses, Ronald Seibold, MS, has discovered:

Through the 1940s and 1950s, cereal grasses were found to contain a number of 'factors' which had different health-related effects on animals. In addition to the growth and fertility factors, grass was shown to contain factors which support the growth of lactobacilli and other beneficial intestinal bacteria.

Cereal grasses contain a factor which blocks the development of scurvy (vitamin C deficiency) which follows the feeding of glucoascorbic acid. This effect could not be duplicated by the feeding of vitamin C (ascorbic acid). Other reports describe a cereal grass factor which blocks the formation of histamine-induced ulcers in guinea pigs. Clinical studies conducted by Dr. Cheney at Stanford in 1950 demonstrated that green vegetables contain a factor which promotes the healing of peptic ulcers.

By 1950, all the nutrients now considered essential to the human diet (with the exception of selenium) had been identified. But researchers continued to describe green food 'factors' which could not be correlated with any known nutrient. In 1957, Ershoff again demonstrated the growth stimulating effect of a green food factor for guinea pigs. All cereal grasses produced similar results…

In 1960, the same laboratory described a water-soluble factor in alfalfa which improved utilization of vitamin A in rats. This factor was shown to be distinct from known nutrients, including the carotenes. In 1966, Dr. George Briggs and others identified a 'plant factor' in grasses, alfalfa and broccoli, which…provided significant growth stimulation when fed to guinea pigs.…To this day the 'Grass Juice Factor' in young green plants, required for life and health in guinea pigs, has still not been identified as any of the known nutrients.

This small bit of information regarding "unknown" factors in foods should tell us two things: First, we must be careful not to be so conceited as to think that our science has outsmarted and surpassed the ancient wisdom of

Mother Nature; and second, that we must recognize that the unknown may be as much of the secret to life and vitality as the known.

Vitamins and minerals and other food constituents are part of a greater whole. As we shall see, not only do vitamins need other cofactors to work, but they also need subfactors. For example, vitamin A needs fat-splitting enzymes, minerals, amino acids and other vitamins for optimum benefit and assimilation. But vitamin A also needs all of its subfactors—not just beta carotene, but also delta carotene, retinal, retinol, and retinoic acid. Similarly, vitamin D and calcium work together. Calcium balances sodium and phosphorus. Vitamin E and selenium are synergists. Vitamin E acts as a cofactor in oxidative phosphorylation reactions; while vitamin C protects vitamin E from oxidation. Riboflavin is a cofactor of thiamin. Choline depends upon folic acid to transfer methyl groups; and choline depends on vitamin B_{12} for its synthesis. The inter workings of vitamins, minerals, amino acids, essential fatty acids, enzymes, coenzymes and other substances are immeasurable. The balance of nutrients is inherent in nature's live foods and is admittedly beyond the full comprehension of man and his limited science. (Shayne, page 15)

THE WISDOM IN NATURE

The wisdom inherent in nature, after all of these millennia, still prevails in promoting health and vitality.

Since deficiencies in vitamins and minerals are known to CAUSE DISEASE AND ILLNESS, then you can see how taking fractions and synthetics may be harmful. If you are suffering from chronic fatigue or stress, for example, your body may be in need of the vitamin B food complex. In such cases, it would be unwise to further deplete your body's store of "real" B vitamins by taking fractionated or synthetic vitamin pills (labeled B1, B3, B6, B12, etc.) either singly or in combination.

It is also important to note that taking a combination of different fractionated vitamins does not equate to taking the same vitamins in a whole food complex supplement. The combination may contain all of the necessary fractions (pieces), but these individual isolates are still lacking the complex arrangement as well as the other components provided by nature to give such vitamins real nutrient value and integrity.

ARE SUPPLEMENTS NECESSARY?

Many doctors tell their patients that they can get all of the vitamins they need from their food, without supplements. This statement is in defiance of the truth about our modern diet which is so depleted, devitalized and altered that real nutrients are just not being consumed in substantial quantity or quality to support human health. The FALSEHOOD of getting your vitamins, minerals and other nutrients from the average modern diet is a ridiculous and antiquated argument befitting a modern medical industry out of touch with (or in denial of) reality. In *HealthxFiles Newsletter* (1997), writer Judith A. DeCava wrote:

> Years ago it was possible to receive all the vitamins, minerals, enzymes, coenzymes and amino acids from our food…exactly where we should get them. However, today we need supplements because:
> - Our soils are depleted of nutrients;
> - Pesticides and synthetic fertilizers poison our foods and environment;
> - Preservatives and other toxic substances are added to commercial foods;
> - Foods are processed, removing essential nutrients to prolong shelf life;

- Our lives are more stressful and fast-paced;
- Fewer raw foods are included in the average diet;
- Foods are being "enriched" with synthetic vitamins and isolated minerals;
- More harmful substances are used: drugs, tobacco, inhalants, aluminum, fluoride, chlorine, nuclear waste;
- Devitalized foods, alcohol, refined carbohydrates and refined sugars are consumed.

Whereas years ago, a patient may have had a few imbalances and/or deficiencies, today's patients have a MULTIPLICITY of complex and serious imbalances or deficiencies. Supplements are used by many natural healthcare doctors to correct these imbalances and deficiencies.

YOU CAN'T FORCE NATURE TO HEAL

Each person is complex and dynamic (ever-changing). Healing takes time, patience and observation to forge ahead in the direction of good health. Nature takes her time; healing is a gradual process of rebuilding. Whole food-complex supplements and good lifestyle habits rebuild the body slowly, NATURALLY, over time without causing an imbalance. The thought of taking supplements as a quick-fix solution to health concerns is medical-thinking, not natural-thinking.

FOODS CAN HEAL

Documented scientific studies have shown that natural, whole foods have been used successfully to heal disease, where fractionated and synthetic vitamins failed to achieve the same results. There are countless books extolling the health benefits of vitamins, ranging from vitamin C to vitamin E. In these books, each vitamin (each a fraction of a whole, natural food) is depicted as having a separate and important function. However, none of these individual vitamins provide a balanced health effect. In analogy, we can say that the spring to a clock has a very definite and important function;

yet we also know that unless this spring remains intact within the clock along with other components, it has no real value in the overall operation and function. When considering the value of a vitamin, it only serves a nutritional purpose while intact in its original food "complex," and not isolated by itself in a vitamin pill. Each vitamin, in its natural complex form, has many functions, including, but not limited to:

- Vitamin A: eyes and skin health; immunity, liver and respiratory/lung health; glandular support
- Vitamin B: nervous system, energy, thinking; heart, liver, glandular health
- Vitamin C: connective tissue; gum and tooth health; wound healing; blood vessel health; respiratory support
- Vitamin D: bone and skeletal health
- Vitamin E: heart and blood vessel health, antioxidant value; reproduction; immunity, glandular support

ARE YOUR VITAMINS REAL?

For a quick comparison of the supplements you may be taking, read the label and consider Dr. Richard Murray's 40 years of biochemical research showing that:

- Vitamin A acetate or palmitate is not vitamin A;
- Beta-carotene is not a carotenoid complex;
- Thiamine hydrochloride or mononitrate is not vitamin B1;
- Pyridoxine hydrochloride is not vitamin B6;
- Niacin is not vitamin B3;
- Ascorbic acid is not vitamin C;
- Irradiated ergosterol is not vitamin D;
- Alpha or mixed tocopherols are not vitamin E.

The body should not be fed these synthetic, fractionated substances in place of whole food complexes which contain the entire range of vitamins plus all of their original cofactors, subfactors, synergists, enzymes and unknown factors. Likewise, don't mistakenly believe that enriched or fortified foods (especially breads and cereals) containing these synthetic substances are any healthier than without them.

HIGH POTENCY

"HIGH POTENCY" is a phrase vitamin manufacturers use to impress people into thinking that man-made chemicals are better than those found in nature. It is not the potency (a word that has been used interchangeably with "strength") that matters, it is the *form* ingested that determines the effect on your body! A potent synthetic vitamin is still not a nutrient. Potency ("strength" measured in micrograms, milligrams, international units, etc.) is one of the criterion used by vitamin manufacturers to standardize dosages of their supplements so that different brands and vitamin products may be compared for presumed effectiveness. Foods found in nature are effective (potent) because of their inherent qualities which are naturally occurring in a "complex," interwoven and naturally balanced state. To synthetically create a super strong (so-called "high potency") substance defies the logic and balance of nature.

WHEN IN DOUBT, TRUST IN NATURE

When in doubt, trust in nature. Vitamins are PARTS of foods, and no longer capable of acting as nutrients when separated from foods and put into pills called "vitamin" supplements. The human body will regard any substance a TOXIN if it is not a food. This has been proven in studies showing the reaction of the body to the introduction of non-food vitamins which create a host of toxic effects on the body ranging from rapid heartbeat, liver damage, skin eruptions, nausea, headaches, fatigue, lowered immunity and failure to rid the body of disease. Even if you consume synthetic or fractionated vitamins and enjoy a pharmacological (drug-like) effect over the course of a few months or so, eventually these substances may deplete the body of its vitality and interfere with normal biochemical functions.

If you take supplements, be sure they are in a live, WHOLE FOOD COMPLEX form. As most doctors will agree, ideally, your vitamins, minerals and other nutrients should come from your diet. But if you eat a typical modern diet, then WHOLE FOOD COMPLEX supplements are biochemically safe, effective and proven by nature to work.

Food researcher Dr. Royal Lee, whose life work in the first half of last century involved using food complexes in the clinical setting, wrote, "The first principle of nutrition is to get ALL the factors needed in the maintenance of the human body. This is unlikely to happen when the nutritional integrity of a vitamin is confused with its chemical integrity."

Perhaps this issue is best summed up in the words of Dr. Judith DeCava, who said, "Nutrition comes from real plants, not from manufacturing plants."

WHAT'S LEFT TO EAT?

Considering all that has been written in the preceding pages regarding toxic foods, artificial ingredients, pesticide residues, organic produce and the impact of eating processed, refined, chemical laden and devitalized foods, you may be thinking, "What's left to eat if I can't sit down at my favorite deli and order a plate of refined pancakes, refined-sugar syrup, pesticide-poisoned coffee, nitrite-laden bacon and glass of milk teeming with hormones and antibiotics?" The answer is simple: Eat what is pure, whole, unaltered and as close to nature as possible. Read labels, avoid chemicals and don't destroy your foods before you consume them.

Every individual has different requirements, genetic traits, personalities, body types, strengths, weaknesses, tastes, metabolisms, immune systems and tolerances. Design your daily diet to suit yourself, because there is no single diet or regimen that is perfect for everyone. Calorie-counting, food pyramids, food combining issues and vitamin and mineral requirements are all theoretical standards that do not take into consideration that we are each individuals. Even members within the same family should have individualized eating, exercise, rest and work habits.

CONCERNED WIVES & MOTHERS

Statistics prove that mothers and wives lead the way in embracing the concept of natural healthcare. They are statistically more open (receptive) than males in accepting ideas in harmony with love and life, and they care enough about their loved ones to search for harmonious solutions.

Alternative Digest magazine (citing *Whole Foods* magazine's 1997 Whole Foods Consumer Survey) reported that the overwhelming majority of those involved in natural healthcare are highly educated women. However, as many experienced practitioners will attest, these women face an uphill battle in winning over their spouses, children and other family members to natural healthcare practices, including improving nutritional standards at home. An intelligent woman may sit in front of her natural healthcare doctor, sigh deeply and exclaim, "What you say about nutrition makes a lot of sense, but what can I do about my husband Rocco? If he doesn't have his roast, his potatoes and a loaf of bread sitting on the table by six o'clock, he gets so irritable that he threatens to kick the cat!" My first word of advice is to tell Rocco to wake up and join the Turn of the Century. The days of making your wife solely responsible for your meals went the way of serfdom. But in all fairness, if you can't convince Rocco to eat more nutritiously, in the least, he should refrain from belittling your positive efforts and stay out of your way to better health.

You cannot force a change of consciousness upon another person, whether that person is your beloved spouse, your dear child or your parents. We are all individuals with something different to learn and to experience, even if that experience is to suffer the effects caused by poor lifestyle and dietary choices. Health consciousness is each individual's choice to pursue or ignore.

GET TO KNOW YOUR HEALTHFOOD STORE

If you are just starting out on the path to greater health, the first step is to find a healthfood store committed to healthy foods (rather than to vitamin pills). When trying to decide which foods to buy, consider your health first then, secondarily, consider taste. Since foods are intended to feed, nourish and build the body, be sure that the foods you buy contain

REAL, whole foods free of other ingredients such as chemicals, bad fats, etc. If there are words on the labels that look like names of chemicals, then avoid them.

What about the higher prices?

What about them? The law of cause and effect is exacting: Your choice is to pay for either good food or for illness. If chemical-laden, toxic foods are your choice, then statistics show that you will pay with your health. "Foul-nutrition" leads to disease that costs you money, time, convenience, mental and emotional stress, worry, and pain. The national cancer rate is rising to 50%, owing mostly to toxic foods and a toxic environment. Tomorrow's disease is more expensive than today's healthiest food bills. If your goal is to buy real foods, then you must pay for them; chemicals and devitalized ingredients are cheaper than foods, which is why so many commercial brand food items seem, by comparison, inexpensive. Your good health is worth the price of real, pure, natural and whole foods which nourish the cells in your body.

READ THE LABELS, READ THE LABELS & READ THE LABELS

One piece of advice goes a long way when shopping even at the health-food store: Read All Labels Carefully! There are a wide number of items on the shelves, some of which are not so healthy, some of which contain too much sugar and some of which contain substitutes for offensive ingredients that are just as bad as the ingredients they are intended to replace. Healthfood store foods can also contain MSG (such as in yellow rice mixtures or seasonings), refined oils, refined sugars and pasteurized juice, just to name a few objectionable items.

A quick checklist…

Read food & supplement labels to avoid:
- All processed and refined foods, including refined sugars and refined flours
- All unnatural preservatives (become familiar with names of chemicals to avoid). You may refer to Ruth Winter's book *Food Additives, Safe Shopper's Bible*, as well as other resources.
- Refined sugar synonyms such as sucrose, corn syrup, fructose, maltose, powdered sugar, glaze, glucose, dextrose, lactose, sorbitol, xylitol, mannitol, caramel, dextrin, polydextrose, invert sugar, high fructose corn syrup, brown sugar, and even often "raw sugar."
- Ingredients you don't understand: Research all ingredients; this is your health we're talking about—don't take chances with chemicals or other artificial ingredients
- Aluminum byproducts and fluoride (an industrial waste by-product); fluoride and aluminum in tooth paste, deodorants, cosmetics, baking powder, tap water, etc.
- All artificial food dyes and colorings
- Pasteurized milk and cheese products; buy organic brands only, but don't expect that these products are a good source of calcium and vitamins, because they are not
- Enriched or fortified foods: These contain synthetic or fractionated (isolated) vitamins not used by the cells as real vitamins. Such so-called vitamins are added to foods and do not contain the entire vitamin "complex"
- Margarine, hydrogenated and/or partially hydrogenated oils, refined oils (even if labeled "cold pressed"). Good oils are unrefined.
- Foods and supplements labeled "natural." The word "natural" is not a guarantee of quality or wholeness, and carries no legal definition or degree of quality to which food and supplement manufacturers must

adhere. By analogy, an arm or a leg is natural, but serves no function unless still attached to the rest of the body.

- Fragmented (isolated) and synthetic vitamins. Purchase either whole food complex supplements that do not contain fragmented vitamins (See Appendix for sources) or avoid buying supplements altogether until you understand the difference.
- Irradiated foods. Irradiated foods are supposed to carry a logo (ask your grocer). To date, only organically grown foods are guaranteed to be non-irradiated. Nuclear waste is now being used as a supposed germ-killer on foods. The result is foods virtually stripped of all their essential nutrients and altered in such a way that many independent scientists claim will lead to increased incidences of cancer and other diseases.

REPLACEMENT FOODS FOR YOUR SHOPPING LIST: HEALTHIER CHOICES FOR BETTER NUTRITION

The following list has been compiled based on consumer and natural prac-titioner feedback. The brand names listed do not imply an endorsement of the particular manufacturer, but only that we have tried that company's products and found them to be a tasty, relatively healthful and reliable alternative to devitalized/chemicalized grocery store brands. The ideal diet is an individual matter and contains natural, whole and pure foods. However, this list provides you with a good base for transition into a healthier lifestyle:

FOOD	REPLACEMENT ITEM
Spaghetti	Preferably organic pastas (healthfood store) such as DeBoles brands; whole wheat, quinoa, corn
Jelly, jams	Organic, sugar-free fruit spreads containing fruits only

Spaghetti sauce	Organic sauce (healthfood store) such as Muir Glen, Enricos, Millenas
Pretzels	Paul Newman, Barbara's brand pretzels
Potato chips	Westbrae's organic potato chips (although any product using heated oil is not recommended)
Cola drinks	Preferably (healthfood store) brands such as Knudsen spritzers
Peanut butter	Arrowhead Mills non-hydrogenated organic
Syrup	Maple syrup (100% pure, organic, no sugars added) or raw honey
Children Cereals	Organic cereals
Salad dressing	Organic brands, or make your own from organic ingredients such as unrefined oil & white wine or apple cider vinegar, Italian seasoning, salt and garlic
Iceberg lettuce	Organic red leaf, green leaf, raw spinach, Romaine
Desserts	Natural, unprocessed pudding; organic fruits; Rice Dream brand (similar to ice cream)
Chocolate	Organic and with unrefined sugar
Salt	Sea Salt
Seasonings	Frontier seasonings, organic, non-irradiated, no preservatives
White sugar	Raw honey or Sucanat, whole sugar cane juice, dehydrated
Salsa	Preferably organic salsa such as Muir Glen, or homemade using organic cilantro, lemon, onion, vinegar, tomato.
Frozen vegetables	Organic, frozen vegetables (Fresh is better); avoid canned vegetables
Catsup	Organic ketchup such as Millena brand
Mustard	Organic yellow or brown mustard
Hamburgers	Free-range organic beef such as Coleman's brand

Cookies	Westbrae organic or Barbara's (organic-only) brand cookies or other organic (healthfood store) alternative; when making your own or buying, avoid refined flour, refined sugar and chemicals
Oil	Extra virgin olive oil, organic and **unrefined** Safflower, sesame seed, sunflower, flaxseed, peanut, etc., Coconut Butter available through Nature's Wellness Center (see Appendix)
Coffee	Organic coffee, bamboo, chicory
Butter/Margarine	Organic (raw if possible) butter, DO NOT USE MARGARINE
Pickles, dill,	Organic brands such as Cascadian Farms sauerkraut
Mayonnaise	Safflower mayonnaise such as Haines, or better yet, homemade
Beef	Free-range, drug-free organic beef, hamburgers, meat, steak, etc.
Hot dogs	Veggie hot dogs or chicken hot dogs (Shelton brand)
Pepperoni	Veggie pepperoni
Chicken	Free-range, organic chicken such as Shelton's brand
Turkey	Free-range, organic turkey such as Diestel brand
Milk	Certified Grade A organic, raw
Cheese	Organic, raw, unpasteurized or at least "natural" cheese. No "cheese food" or processed cheeses
Juices	Organic, such as Mountain Sun brand; freshly-made/squeezed juices from organic fruits & vegetables is best because most other juices are heated or pasteurized, destroying vitamins and enzymes
Nuts	Raw, organic and NOT ROASTED
Spreads	Nut butters: sesame (tahini), almond, cashew, apple
Chocolate milk	Amazake (Grainaissance) or unrefined cocoa powder with Certified Grade A organic raw milk

Bread	Organic bread or at least whole grain bread from health food store
SOAP	For showering, washing: liquid castile soap, such as Dr. Bronner's brand
DEODORANT	Natural only, do not use aluminum-based antiperspirants; find herbal varieties
FLUORIDE	Avoid fluoride in foods, water and at the dentist.
CHLORINE	Buy a chlorine shower filter to avoid absorption of chlorine through the skin and by inhaling the steam.
WATER	Do not drink or cook with tap water. Look into installing a reverse osmosis system at the kitchen sink as well as a whole house water purification/ filer system.
SUPPLEMENTS	Avoid most store bought vitamins, especially "high potency." Use whole food complex supplements only from a reliable manufacturer such as NutriPlex Formulas, Inc.. Avoid being fooled by the word "natural". Do not be lured into supplement fads. Avoid multivitamins and mineral concoctions, as well as amino acid supplements.

READ ALL LABELS on every product before you purchase it to avoid chemicals, preservatives, synthetic and isolated vitamins ("enriched" foods), pesticides, aluminum, dyes, colorings, artificial ingredients, artificial flavoring, emulsifiers, hydrogenated and/or partially hydrogenated oils, refined sugars such as sucrose, fructose, refined white sugar, brown sugar, high fructose corn syrup, corn syrup.

CORPORATIONS & INSTITUTIONS SHAPING OUR HEALTH & EATING DECISIONS
& PERSPECTIVES ON ATTITUDE & AWARENESS

Each physical condition we face is somehow related to our state of consciousness—our state of awareness of life—which leads us to experience the effect of the choices we make. Our nonphysical selves expressed as our thoughts, attitudes, feelings, intuition, emotions and actions—positive or negative—are manifested into our physical states of being. Therefore, health is as much a spiritual state of existence as it is a physical state of being. Our state of health is affected by our choices. Choices begin at the point of intent. Therefore, the way we think, the way we look at things, is the most important determining factor of our health, now and in the future.

Unless we learn and practice the art of conscious living—living wisely in a state of awareness of the interplay of life in all of its complexities—we are destined to live like a speck of dust in the wind, being blown around without taking control over our own destiny. Without eating and living consciously, we forfeit our power and control over our own destiny to someone or something outside of ourselves; then we become the effect of their thoughts, willpower, emotions and actions. Besides creating problems for ourselves, such an approach to living is at best irresponsible. And irresponsibility creates negative (undesirable) effects that lead to suffering.

Once we train ourselves to recognize how we will be affected in all situations, we can then begin to take control over our health and awaken to the fact that disease, degeneration and death is less the result of some inevitable, "unlucky" process, but rather more the result of our lack of conscious awareness that guides us into taking the wisest actions.

In a world full of sick people, it is difficult for the average person to conceive of the fact that sickness is rarely something that just happens TO us. Rather, illness is most usually the result of absent-minded actions. It's the difference between eating eating organic foods and not, between eating refined sugars vs. unrefined, between inhaling toxic fumes rather than using a non-toxic alternative, and between eating junk food full of chemical ingredients vs. eating snack foods without any chemicals. Since "everybody's doing it," people rarely take the time to investigate healthier choices in food, sprays, paints, supplements, healthcare, cosmetics, person hygiene products, water, air and foods.

What makes chemical-laden foods and toxic products the "norm"? The answer is: manufacturers who successfully convince the public of the health and safety of their deadly, cancer- and disease-causing products. With greater awareness, thankfully, the general public is slowly beginning to wake up and smell the carrot juice. The burgeoning healthfood and natural products industries are proof of this trend. The net result is a healthier population who has taken notice that there IS A CHOICE.

WHO'S CONTROLLING YOUR CHOICES?

How aware are you of the influences motivating you to purchase certain products or eat certain foods? Are you in control of your decisions, or do you surrender them to corporations more interested in their profit margins than your well-being? Most people have very little understanding of how their bodies work and what they need to eat to live in health. It is also true that poor eating habits are reinforced by corporations bombarding us with false, but convincing, messages promising benefits unsubstantiated by biochemical fact. Or, we are given partial facts about foods which do not apply to the food that ends up in our refrigerators. For instance, from the time a mineral-rich potato is pulled from the soil to the time it ends up in a bag of potato chips, its nutritional integrity has been destroyed. An orange may start off as a great source of vitamin C, but by the time it is drenched with pesticides and synthetic fertilizers then pasteurized and brought to your grocery store, it is a substance no longer resembling its original natural form. Its enzymes are destroyed as well as its original vitamin C content.

Does milk "do a body good," as television commercials tell us? If you live on a farm or are fortunate enough to be able to purchase and drink certified Grade A raw milk, then yes, milk can do you good. But the truth is that almost all milk sold to the public is pasteurized, which results in the alteration and destruction of enzymes, vitamins, amino acids, essential fats and other nutrients needed to support cellular health.

But that's not all. It has taken a powerful, persistent marketing campaign to get Americans to eat more meat than anyone else on the planet— 246 pounds a year for every man, woman and child. Is meat really that bad? Again, the answer falls into the "yes-and-no" category. Meat, poultry and dairy can be a viable food choice, but not when livestock are raised on toxic feed, injected with hormones, antibiotics and other drugs and raised in environments breeding insanity, torture, stress and cancer. The healthiest sources of these foods are "free-range," organically grown varieties (the way animals were raised in the past) now found in many healthfood stores. And the ideal way to eat them is by only marginally cooking them to prevent the fragile complex of nutrients from being altered and destroyed.

INFLUENCING OUR CHILDREN AT SCHOOL & AT HOME

John Robbins, author of *Diet for A New America* (71), tells us that recommendations for eating, as supplied through the school system by dairy farmers, are biased. Such recommendations make it "hard to avoid the perception that the [dairy industry] is primarily concerned with getting youngsters hooked on high-fat dairy products, and that providing sound nutritional education to children is merely a pretext."

Robbins postulates: "Could part of the reason so many of us struggle with unhealthy food habits be that when we were young, vulnerable, and impressionable, we were 'educated' by materials such as these?"

A half hour in front of the television set during Saturday morning (or after-school) cartoons is proof enough to anyone that "food" commercials aimed at children are manipulative enough to make cookies and milk seem like a logical choice for breakfast. And if you take your children through the aisles of today's supermarket, you'll quickly discover how influential such commercials are in creating a demand for cookies, cakes, candies, cereals, dairy products, soft drinks, snack foods and so on, as your children recognize and request familiar brand names and packaging. Corporate giants have dug their claws into the growing minds of our children without any remorse or hesitation or consideration of the effects.

Children in our modern era of devitalized and processed foods are suffering, and the media is reluctant, due to pressures by their sponsors and owners, to expose the serious and widespread ill effects. It would even be accurate to say that the media is a major causative factor in the demise of health in this country.

Dr. Carl Jensen (72) writes, "Kaiser Permanente Department of Allergy chief emeritus, Ben F. Feingold [M.D.], hypothesized in 1973 that one to five million American school children diagnosed as hyperkinetic [hyperactive] are actually victims of toxicity due to ingestion of artificially dyed and flavored foods. One hundred 'Feingold Associations' claimed great success by applying these findings."

In clinical practice, we have witnessed remarkable results with behaviorally, and so-labeled "psychologically" troubled, children by simply feeding them real nutrition. A lack of real foods, combined with a diet of artificial, processed and synthetically "enriched" foods, is a recipe for a host of illnesses so numerable that we have not yet come close to identifying them all. Children are not growing unruly, hyperactive and unable to focus on a single thought as the result of some stupefying genetic trait, but rather from a lack of significant food factors which are absolutely required by the cells in their bodies to provide biochemical function. Dr. Jensen explains, "research over the past 15 years has shown the right foods, or the natural neurochemicals they contain, can enhance mental capabilities." To take Jensen's statement further, it can be said that such foods are in fact REQUIRED for mental capabilities and brain development.

Do you think for a moment that food giants who support television with their multi-billion-dollar advertising contracts will allow the television networks to report the hazards of foul-nutrition creating ill-health in our children (as well as the rest of us)? This will never happen unless one day the corporate giants seek an audience with the Wizard of Oz to infuse them with a conscience.

HYPERACTIVE, ATTENTION DEFICIT DISORDERED CHILDREN: WHO'S CALLING IT A 'DISEASE'?

Robert Mendelsohn, M.D., makes us wonder about the "epidemic" of hyperactive children saddled with the invented disease called Attention Deficit Disorder (ADD). He writes (p. 33-34):

> No modern medical procedure better displays the inquisitorial nature of Modern Medicine than the drugging of so called "hyperactive" children. Originally, behavior controlling drugs were used to treat only the most severe cases of mental illness. But today, drugs such as Dexedrine, Cylert, Ritalin, and Tofranil are being used on more than a million children through the Unite States—on the basis of often flimsy diagnostic criteria of hyper activity and minimal brain damage. Some medical tests, when performed correctly. But there is no single diagnostic test that will identify a child

as hyperactive or any of the twenty-one other names assigned to this syndrome. The list of inconclusive tests is at least as long as the list of names. All a doctor has to go on is a list of inconclusive tests and the "educated" guess of an "expert."

One school in Texas took advantage of this ambiguity and diagnosed forty percent of its students as minimal brain damaged in a year when government money was available to treat the syndrome. Two years later, this money was no longer available, but funds for treating children with language learning disabilities were floating around. Suddenly, the minimally brain damaged students disappeared and thirty-five percent of the children were diagnosed as having language learning disabilities!

…the child who can't sit still in class—instead of being given tasks that will occupy him—is diagnosed as hyperactive and "managed" by drugs. These drugs are not without serious side effects. Not only do they suppress growth and cause high blood pressure, nervousness, and insomnia, but they transform children into "brave new world" type zombies. Sure, the kids slow down—dramatically. They're also less responsive and enthusiastic, and more humorless and apathetic. And they don't perform any better when measured objectively over long periods of time.

GROWING UP ON WRONG IMPRESSIONS

How would your child deduce that a candy bar is harmful to her health when TV ads tout its "benefits" by announcing, "Rough day? Smooth it out with a Milky Way!" And what can be gleaned from the Snickers candy bar commercials exclaiming, "Hungry? Why wait?" In one Saturday morning commercial for a popular children's sugary cereal, the announcer authoritatively proclaims, "It tastes so good, who cares about anything else?" Do you care? I do, but apparently not the cereal company that is cleverly deceitful enough to refer to refined sugar as "frosting." Such manufacturers are covering up the fact that refined sugar/processed cereals are no good for the consumer and are engineered primarily to taste good to increase sales and gain consumer loyalty. Health is not an issue to be trifled with.

A child who is bombarded by clever, powerful, purposeful and persuasive advertising messages is taught from an early age that taste takes precedence over nutrition when it comes to food choices.

According to Phyllis Herman, CNS, MS (*Health News & Review*, 1995: 12), "when children choose their foods from among those touted on Saturday morning TV, they are eating mostly non-nutritive junk foods rich in fat and sugar like fast foods, candy, chips, sodas and sugar-coated cereals."

Generation after generation is brought up on television, the most powerful force shaping our public opinion and perception of truth, sweeping us further and further from nature and Her bounty as our bodies suffer with illness at an alarming rate. Further, this worldwide rise in disease goes unreported on the same media which is owned and directed by the very powers creating chemical concoctions that they strive to convince us is really food.

SWITCHING KIDS TO ORGANIC FOODS

Jennifer Bogo, *E Magazine*, (*E Magazine*, March/April 2001, pp. 42-44) writes:
    Pesticide residues on conventional kids' food continues to be too high, according to a follow-up to the 1999 Consumers' Union report "Do You Know What You're Eating?" Close scrutiny of five years' worth of data from the U.S. Department of Agriculture's Pesticide Data Program demonstrated that the safe chronic dose of chemicals, the level at which the Environmental Protection Agency feels "reasonably certain" a child would suffer no harm over

lifetime exposure, was exceeded with several foods. And while the report's authors calculate that the odds of any single child getting an acute dose of pesticides are small, odds that a dangerous dose will reach a significant number across the whole population, 20 million U.S. children age six or younger, are great. Especially when adding up exposures from multiple foods and meals.

...One million kids under six exceed their safe chronic dose on any given day. And more than 63 daily exposures to persistent...pollutants (linked to serious developmental disorders) are likely, according to the Pesticide Action Network's "Nowhere to Hide" report released this past November [2000].

"The more we learn about chemicals in the environment, the more we learn that very, very early in life is the most susceptible period," says Dr. Gina Solomon of the Natural Resources Defense Council. Childhood is a period of critical organ development and rapid growth. And during this vulnerable time, children pound-for-pound ingest more food and drink more water than adults, and have less diverse diets, exposing them to more concentrated residues.

The good news is that the organic foods industry is on the rise, fueled by intelligent, savvy and caring parents. From infancy, it is entirely possible for parents to raise their children on organic, healthy foods, from baby foods to children's cereals. Companies such as Stonyfield Farms, Healthy Times, Yo Baby, Whole Kids, and others are providing drug-free, chemical-free, organic baby foods, snack foods and yogurt. "Organic companies are scrambling to assure the parents of growing kids that even processed foods like pop tarts and pudding snacks can be made from healthy ingredients, while still appealing to the sensibilities of their younger, and more finicky, market," Bogo writes.

The children's market for organic foods is experiencing considerable growth as a result of parental demand, according to Paddy Spence, CEO of San Francisco-based Spence Information Services. "Take dairy, for instance: In the last year, organic milk sales have increased more than 40 percent in natural food stores, and yogurt, more than 45. Such growth can be seen in conventional supermarkets too. [Not just healthfood stores]. Fourteen percent of parents polled by Hartman's Organic Lifestyle Shopper Study during 2000 say they buy organics and natural foods for kids under age 18; the same is true for 20 percent of parents with kids under age six."

Thanks to consumer demand, "grab-and-go" foods are gaining popularity as well. Pavich, a major player in organic foods, has introduced snack packs of 100 percent natural, organic raisins; Happy Herberts offers organic pretzel sticks, and, writes Bogo:

> [Planet Harmony] now boasts organic jelly beans, fruit snacks and gummy worms; Country Choice Naturals, organic animal cookies; Organic Foods, Inc., soy pops (much like Kix); and Earthbound Farms, serving sized organic carrot sticks and salad bags, with all natural dressing. For putting together those PB&J sandwiches, Alvarado St. Bakery offers the Ultimate Kids Bread, baked from organic whole wheat flours and sweetened with local honey..Organic juices, too, fit in little lunch boxes for a no-mess drink. RW Knudsen has organic apple juice, and Santa Cruz, organic grape, lemon, orange and tropical flavors.

Other foods, including Environ-Kidz cereal, are backed by education on organic foods and endangered species, and at least one percent of sales are donated to environmental and children's charities.

The bottom line is that foul-nutrition is, by popular demand spurred by an awareness of the awful composition of children's foods, being replaced with real nutrition by parents who understand the dangers of refined, chemical and pesticide-laden foul nutrition. Ultimately, however, the next step after switching over to organic choices in packaged foods is to begin to introduce more and more raw fruits, vegetables, seeds, nuts and juices into the diet. Kids should not only be able to taste carrot juice, but they should be taught in school as well as at home to appreciate its nutrient-dense qualities for supporting health and vitality. At this point in the evolution of our schools and teaching methodology, children are at best learning about real foods while being rewarded with cake, cookies and candy. This sends conflicting messages to very impressionable children who are just forming their opinions of right and wrong and good and bad.

EXPLOITING THE NATION THROUGH ADVERTISING

While parents are beginning to see the light and making dietary corrections at home, corporations and educators are thwarting their efforts at school, where children spend most of their day.

Nutrition Action Healthletter (January/February 2001) reports:

> Because corporations don't respect boundaries…we fear they'll turn our homes into showrooms for pitchmen, our schools into amphitheaters for marketing, and our national parks into billboard showcases." And children are now becoming prime targets. "Corporations used to respect the fact that children are precious beings to be nurtured," says Gary Ruskin, [director of Commercial Alert, a non-profit group in Washington, DC, that opposes excesses in commercialism, advertising, and marketing]. "Now under pressure to increase profits, many corporations see kids as economic resources to be exploited, like raw timber or bauxite. Many parents fear that corporations will turn our kids into smoking, drinking, violence-loving, obese addicts."
>
> Even schools don't offer refuge. More than 12,000 of them subscribe to Channel One, a daily commercial television news program broadcast by satellite. "These schools

force their children to sit and watch commercials for fast foods and soft drinks, the very kinds of foods that are making them fatter," says Ruskin. And not just fatter. Ads push foods like burgers, fries, pizza and ice cream...all prepping our kids and teens for a lifetime of gridlocked arteries and steadily rising blood pressure.

"There's been such a dramatic increase in advertising and corporate power of the past three decades that many of us have a growing sense that the relentless creep of commercialism threatens much of what makes life worth living," says Ruskin.

Food marketing and advertising have increased dramatically in recent years. From 1988, the number of dollars spent for soft drink advertising rose by 28 percent, for candy and snacks by 40 percent, and for restaurants by 86 percent. The U.S. food industry is the second largest advertiser (the auto industry is number one).

U.S. Department of Agriculture figures show that the proportion of advertising money that companies spend on candy and snacks, prepared convenience foods, and soft drinks far exceeds these foods' share of the American diet. What the food industry spends just on promoting snacks and nuts matches the entire USDA's budget for nutrition research, education and other activities.

"Twenty corporations pay for nearly three-quarters of all food advertising in the U.S.," says Ronald Cotterrill, professor of marketing at the University of Connecticut. "And they spend it to promote highly processed foods like soft drinks, cookies and convenience foods."

USING THE NEWS MEDIA FOR WEALTH OVER HEALTH

Having dismissed cultures of the Far East, as well as their philosophies and healing systems as "unscientific nonsense," Western society, drowning in our own ethnocentricity, owes most of its thoughts and beliefs regarding healthcare to financially motivated pharmaceutical concerns, corporate farming coalitions, food processors, chemical companies and other industrial giants who fully understand the selfish benefit in controlling, defining and setting the boundaries for "accepted" forms of healthcare practices and eating choices in our "civilized" world. Their advertising and marketing campaigns are relentless.

According to John Robbins (12), "Entire industries are focused on maintaining the illusion that we can be happy, well-fed and 'real' only if we consume their products. Remarkably, these forces beset us not only through advertisements, marketing campaigns and other obvious efforts to control our food choices for commercial purposes. Their agendas are also found frequently, and with dire consequences, in classrooms, in governmental agencies, and in hospitals."

WHO'S DEFINING A 'HEALTHY DIET'?"
POLITICAL CONNECTIONS BEHIND THE SCENES

When you understand the politics of modern healthcare, it becomes clear how common sense flies out the window in the face of the almighty dollar. We have only to look at who finances educational materials, university studies and policies to discover why hospital nutrition and dietitians' advice too often promotes unhealthy diets. Due to the political and financial ties to processed food manufacturers and chemical producers, many dietitians and medical doctors are slowly breaking away from the many falsehoods and misinformation that influence perceptions about healthy foods.

The news media have ignored and refused to report the fact that hospitals and schools across the United States have allowed fast food restaurants such as McDonald's to take up residence as the institution's official dining room. You don't have to go down the block for a burger and fries because the restaurant is now right there IN the hospital itself, replacing the cafeteria. How much credibility does such flagrant violation of common sense give medical doctors, dietitians and hospital administrators who are preaching to the public that they understand nutrition, are interested in patient recovery and support a healthy community?

New York Times columnist Marian Burros wrote (Nov. 15, 1995, The Living Section): "The stated mission of the American Dietetic Association, the country's largest professional organization of dietitians, is 'to improve the health of the public.' But the group, which has more than 65,000 members and influences the public through its Consumer Nutrition Hotline, its publications and its nationwide network of spokesmen who are widely quoted on nutrition matters, is being increasingly criticized for its aggressive pursuit of cash and in-kind contributions from trade groups like the Sugar Association and the National Livestock and Meat Board and from individual companies like Coca-Cola, M&M Mars, McDonald's and Sara Lee." Ms Burros reminds us of the American Dietetic Association's most fundamental position: "There are no good or bad foods," and tells us that this "is a wishy-washy stance that derives from industry money...Joan Gussow, a former head of the nutrition education program at Teachers College at Columbia University, says the American Dietetic Association's reliance on industry money means that 'they never criticize the food industry.'"

Dietitians, who are responsible for nutritional advice in hospitals and the school system, among others, are often restricted by their association's political/economic ties. As such, dietitians are found endorsing—and refuse to take a stand against—MacDonald's and other fast foods, chocolate, bovine growth hormone, olestra, candy bars, soda, genetic engineering, genetic modification of foods, and margarine. The National Association of Margarine Manufacturers, which supports the dietetic association with grant money, claims "There is little scientific evidence to suggest that current consumption levels of trans-fatty acids need to be changed." But, according to Marion Burros, "Dr. Walter Willett, the chairman of the department of nutrition at Harvard University, takes vigorous exception. 'There is clear evidence from well-controlled studies that trans-fatty acids, at levels consumed by Americans, have important adverse effects on blood cholesterol fractions, sufficient to account for approximately 30,000 premature deaths a year.'" There is NOTHING natural about margarine.

With a little understanding of the political and economic foundation beneath the advice of the medical and dietetic community, it becomes clear how dietitians monitoring meals in schools and hospitals advocate the serving of sugar-filled gelatin desserts, cola drinks and chocolate cake. These healthcare professionals are entrusted to understand the effects of consuming such deleterious substances in the recovery process from surgery and illness. The last thing a patient expects is to be fed non-foods while sitting in his/her hospital bed!

MONOPOLIZING THE HEALTHCARE INDUSTRY

The natural healthcare industry is regarded as a threat to the modern medical healthcare industry. There is an ongoing campaign by the modern medical establishment, fueled by pharmaceutical companies, to curtail the activity of vitamin and supplement manufacturers, nutritionists, alternative healthcare practitioners, medical doctors practicing alternative healthcare, practitioners of Traditional Chinese Medicine and Ayurvedic medicine, healthfood stores and chiropractic physicians. The pharmaceutical companies and American Medical Association lobby diligently to take away our individual rights to our choice of healthcare and the products we take. There is a move to establish medical doctors and registered dietitians as the sole health practitioners in this country so that all others lose their right to suggest alternative solutions to illness or to practice nutrition. The American Medical Association, American Dietetic Association and pharmaceutical manufacturers are attempting to create legislation that exempt all healthcare providers except medical doctors from dispensing vitamins and supplements, offering professional health advice and treating patients. These institutions apply constant pressure on the FDA to redefine standards for healthcare and the types of substances which should be "approved" for our individual use, such as herbs, vitamins, minerals, enzymes, lotions, creams, etc. All of the activities aimed against natural healthcare are disguised as measures "for the public good," yet the only outcome is loss of freedom to choose one's course of healthcare, treatment, and supplements. So each time you read in the newspaper about the potential "dangers" of supplements and natural healthcare, be sure to consider the source; and consider the very real dangers of drugs, surgeries, injections, laser treatments and ignorance of nutrition. Don't let politics get in the way of your healthcare choices. When a controversy arises over foods and substances such as olestra, Nutrasweet™, or MSG, consider the economic motivation for any group who supports such unhealthy foul-nutrition.

And if you find yourself in a hospital, have your relatives bring you some real food. Julian Whitaker, MD (*Health & Healing* 1995) tells us:

> Malnutrition in hospitals is so rampant that an estimated 50,000 patients starve to death each year. In 1984, *Forbes* magazine described hospital malnutrition as 'staggering,' and it hasn't improved at all...According to a 1988 review of hospital malnutrition studies by Alice Smith, MS, RD, 75% of people who were well-nourished on admission to hospitals became malnourished after only two weeks. When nutritional support was given, an unbelievable 95% received it only after they had developed complications!... Yet if you bring in some nutritional supplements to a hospitalized family member, you are often blocked by the hospital Registered Dietitian, who along with conventional physicians, is responsible for 'staggering' hospital malnutrition.

Pediatrician/author Robert Mendelsohn, M.D., (pp. 85-86) agrees, advising:

If you expect to survive your hospital stay without starving, you have to take responsibility for your own nutrition. If the hospital food is not up to your standards, you should have it brought in from home. (if the hospital food *is* up to your standards, either you're in an exceptional hospital or you should seriously reexamine your dietary habits).

BIG MONEY IN INVENTING DISEASES

How are diseases created? Some doctors say it's germs, while others claim toxic poisoning. Still others say diseases are caused by poor diets lacking vital nutrients. But here's a new way of creating disease that has become very popular these days: Diseases can be created by just giving symptoms a name. For instance, television commercials being played as of this writing (2001) are now telling us that women experiencing premenstrual symptoms of bloating, mood swings and discomfort are stricken with a disease called PMDD (premenstrual dysphoric disorder). It's just a new name for an old problem. Lisa Belkin, in her article "Prime Time Pushers," (*Mother Jones*, March/April 2001, p. 35) explains:

> One television ad that I find particularly egregious, bordering on offensive, is for a relatively new drug called Sarafem. The chemical composition of the pill is identical to that of Prozac, but last summer manufacturer Eli Lilly and Company received FDA permission to market it simultaneously for treatment of premenstrual disphoric disorder, or PMDD. The condition differs from PMS in that its symptoms are [supposedly] more emotional than physical and include depression, anxiety and bursts of anger. And yet a television spot for the drug shows a frustrated woman struggling with a shopping cart in front of a supermarket, and makes Sarafem look like an easy fix for your average bad day.

"They're making everything into a disease, adds Dr. Nash [Ira S. Mash, M.D., associate director of the cardio-vascular institute at the Mount Sinai School of Medicine, New York], "and not only is it a disease, but it's a disease that society has a pill for."

By referring to this problem as a DISEASE, however, pharmaceutical companies and doctors can now sell more drugs. It's as simple as that: To make more money, just invent a disease for the purpose of selling more drugs, including vaccines and flu shots. This practice is more common that most people realize, as more and more diseases are being invented every day, from the Hanta Virus to Chronic Fatigue Syndrome, from the Asian flu to Attention Deficit Disorder (ADD).

Many "medical insiders" would go so far to say that ethics and scientific research are not bedfellows. When it comes to drug and disease studies, investors want to see "results." These results become the bases for "proving" the efficacy and value of drugs and therapies, as well as disease causation. Robert Mendelsohn, M.D., (pp. 124-126) recounts:

> The dean of Harvard Medical School, Dr. Robert H. Ebert, and the dean of the Yale Medical School, Dr. Lewis Thomas, acted as paid consultants to the Squibb Corporation at the same time they were trying to persuade the Food and Drug Administration to lift the ban on Mysteclin, one of Squibb's biggest moneymakers. Dr. Ebert said that he "gave the best advice I could. These were honest opinions." But he also declined to specify the amount of the "modest retainer" Squibb Vice-President Norman R. Ritter admitted paying both him and Dr. Thomas. Dr. Ebert later became a paid director of the drug company and admitted to owning stock valued at $15,000.
>
> In 1972, Dr. Samuel S. Epstin, then of Case-Western Reserve University, one of the world's authorities on chemical causes of cancer and birth defects, told the Senate

Select Committee on Nutrition and Human Needs that "the National Academy of Sciences is riddled with conflict of interest." He reported that panels that decide on crucial issues such as safety of food additives frequently are dominated by friends or direct associates of the interests that are supposed to be regulated. In this country you can buy the data you require to support your case" he said.

Fraud in scientific research is commonplace enough to keep it off the front pages. The Food and Drug Administration has uncovered such niceties as overdosing and underdosing of patients, fabrication of records, and drug dumping when they investigate experimental drug trials. Of course, in these instances, doctors working for drug companies have as their goal producing results that will convince the FDA to approve the drug. Sometimes, with competition for grant money getting more and more fierce, doctors simply want to produce results that will keep the funding lines open. Since all the "good ol' boy" researchers are in the same boat, there seems to be a great tolerance for sloppy experiments, unconfirmable results, and carelessness in interpreting results.

Dr. Ernest Borke, a University of Colorado microbiologist, said that "increasing amounts of faked data or, less flagrantly, data with *body English* put on them, make their way into scientific journals." Nobel Price winner Salvatore E. Luria, a biologist at he Massachusetts Institute of Technology, said "I know of at least two cases in which highly respected scientists had to retract findings reported from their laboratories, because they discovered that these findings had been manufactured by one of their collaborators."

Dr. Mendelsohn continues:

> Of course, research fraud is nothing new. Cyril Burt, the late British psychologist who became famous for his claims that most human intelligence is determined by heredity, was exposed as a fraud by Leon Kamin, a Princeton psychologist...There is even evidence that Gregor Mendel, father of the gene theory of heredity, may have doctored the results of his pea-breeding experiments to make them conform more perfectly to his theory. Mendel's conclusions *were* correct, but a statistical analysis of his published data shows that the odds were 10,000 to one against their having been obtained through experiments such as Mendel performed.

There are many many accusations of fraud, error, misinterpretation and "massaging" of the truth involved in medical and scientific research. The troubling part of all of this is, of course, the fact that the victims of bad research are consumers, patients and the public at large. Who, for instance, pays the ultimate price for dangerous drugs? And who suffers for being kept ignorant of the marvels of proper nutrition and healthy lifestyle choices?

VIRUSES AND BACTERIA: A SMOKE SCREEN?

Confessions of a Medical Heretic, by Robert S. Mendelsohn, M.D., is so full of the cold truth that it'll send shivers up your spine. Although his work may seem at first like a negative attack on the medical profession, his experience as a physician, combined with his research, confirms our innermost suspicions about what is truly health-promoting and the parts of modern medicine that threaten our health and vitality. Dr. Mendelsohn explains the politics of modern medicine (Mendelsohn, 121) by making an analogy to a new "religion" that is complete with its own god, priests, churches and rituals. His description within the analogy stimulates us into thinking that the modern medical paradigm both creates a buffer between the patient and the doctor, and wages a holy war against all other modes of healing and health professions:

> When a new religion wants to discredit an old religion, it does so by blaming the problems of the people on the old gods. Modern Medicine says your disease is caused by a virus. Who created the virus? The old God. And so on. It's not you or we who are causing your disease, it's natural things such as viruses and bacteria and the tendency of cells to divide irregularly and heredity and…The old God is responsible—the God of Life.

> Modern Medicine can free you from the bonds of the old God. Modern Medicine can give you a new God that can counteract all the pesky forms of life that get in the way, such as bacteria, viruses, cells dividing out of control, inconvenient fetuses, deformed or retarded children, and old people.

Dr. Mendelsohn's explanation amounts to this philosophy: Modern medicine has proposed to us that what is natural is evil, including bacteria, viruses, herbs, food cures and naturalism and spiritualism. These have all been replaced by the new God—the one bearing a prescription pad in one hand and a surgical scalpel in the other. Under the "new religion" of modern medicine, the expression of natural healthcare is made to be blasphemy.

IS THE THREAT OF HIV AN INVENTED DISEASE SAID TO CAUSE AIDS?

It has even been stated by the world's leading AIDS researcher, virologist Dr. Peter Duesberg, that AIDS caused by "HIV infection" is also an invention borne of politics and economics that made one particular pharmaceutical company and the inventor of the drug AZT more than a billion dollars in earnings. (Read *Inventing the AIDS Virus*, Dr. Peter Duesberg). Duesberg (601) writes:

> Fascinated by the past triumphs of the germ theory, the public, science journalists, and even scientists from other fields never question the authority of their medical experts, even if they fail to produce useful results (Adams, 1989; Schwitzer, 1992). Medical scientists are typically credited for the virtual elimination of infectious diseases with vaccines and antibiotics, although most of the credit for eliminating infectious diseases is actually owed to vastly improved nutrition and sanitation...Indeed, the belief in the infallibility of modern science is the only ideology that unifies the 20th century. For example, in the name of the virus-AIDS hypothesis of the American government and American researcher Gallo, antibody-positive Americans have been convicted for "assault with a deadly weapon" because they had sex with antibody-negatives, Central Africa dedicates its limited resources to "AIDS testing," the former U.S.S.R. conducted 20.2 million AIDS tests in 1990 and 29.4 million in 1991 to identify a total of 178 antibody-positive Soviets and communists Cuba even quarantines its own citizens if they are antibody-positive...

> Predictably, the AIDS virus hunters, on their last crusade for the germ theory, have no regard for the current drug-use epidemic and its many overlaps with American and European AIDS. Even direct evidence for the role of drugs in AIDS is fiercely rejected by the virus-AIDS orthodoxy... Merely questioning the therapeutic or prophylactic benefits of AZT is protested by the AIDS establishment...The prejudice against noninfectious pathogens is so popular that he virus-AIDS establishment uses it regularly to intimidate

those who propose noninfectious alternatives, to censor
their papers…and even to question their integrity…

As the leading researcher on AIDS, Duesberg discovered and reported
that HIV does not actually cause AIDS, not that AIDS does not exist.
Neither is his work a refutation of the sincere and dedicated work of those
campaigning for a cure for the disease. Duesberg's 700-page book is the
culmination of years of research and proof, for which he lost his job,
research grant and credibility due to the threat that his work presented to
drug companies and medical institutions profiting from the disease.

Similarly, researchers such as Ralph W. Moss, Ph.D., have lost their
jobs and status by reporting the benefits and successes of natural substances in the fight against cancer and other diseases. Dr. Moss says, upon
discovering the benefits of laetrile (an extract made from apricot kernels)
against cancer, "I was instructed to lie about the outcome of our studies. It
became a major cover-up" despite the fact that "one of the outstanding
cancer scientists in the world had shown that it [laetrile] did work to a certain degree." Says Moss, the **official** position of Memorial Sloan Kettering
Cancer Center (one of the most prestigious cancer research institutions in
the world) was that laetrile studies on cancer were negative. Moss explains:

> …Dr. Thomas, president of the Center, along with Drs.
> Good, Old, and Stock—all important scientists [who are
> all M.D.s]—went to Washington, DC, in 1974, and again
> in 1975, to argue the case for laetrile and to urgently request
> permission to conduct clinical trials. The Food and Drug
> Administration…—at that time allied with the American
> Cancer Society and the National Cancer Institute—turned
> them down flat. The upshot was that if Sloan-Kettering was
> going to continue to **receive government and foundation
> funding**, it had better back off on the issue of laetrile,
> which it immediately did…
>
> I held a press conference at the New York Hilton…and
> revealed what I knew about laetrile. I was fired from Sloan-

Kettering the next day. (Mason, *Alternative Complementary Therapies*: 21-22)

If the notion of inventing disease, as well as corporate cover-up and deceit, sounds like science fiction to you, then the pharmaceutical manufacturers have successfully done their job of selling you on their propaganda. Real scientists with outstanding credentials lose their jobs, research grants, reputations and livelihoods by reporting the truth about whether diseases are real or invented for the purpose of selling more drugs and funding institutions for "research" that will never lead to a discovery. There's too much money to lose by exposing the truth about disease, drugs, chemicals, industrial waste and alternative therapies. Even the movie industry has been addressing the subject matter, with films such as Erin Brockevich, Silkwood, Conspiracy Theory, The Fugitive, and others, to mirror the problems of corporate cover-ups, espionage and invention commonplace in our country.

DISEASES ARE GOOD FOR BUSINESS

Groups such as cancer, asthma and heart societies have been around for decades without even coming close to curing their respective diseases despite the billions of dollars **given to them** by donations from real, hardworking people whose lives have been deeply touched by the diseases. Where do the donations for research and prevention go? I have personally seen hundreds of thousands of dollars spent at local banquets funded by these societies to present accolades to doctors for "the fine work they are doing," yet for the real people—those suffering with disease and their family members— there is little or no progress made. Finding a cure would be bad for business, for without finding a cure, such associations continue to thrive, giving jobs and money to doctors, "researchers," scientists, writers, public relations practitioners, hospitals, hospices, universities, laboratories, publishers, support groups and drug companies.

Diseases are BIG business. The more diseases that can be invented, the more money can be made. It's a matter of business for the drug companies, hospitals, universities, advertisers and associations, but for us it's a personal matter of life and death; health and vitality.

The truth is that most research on diseases in this country never results in a cure! And disease research focuses on drugs, viruses, bacteria and genetics, not nutrients in foods because research is funded by drug and chemical companies, not organic farmers dedicated to naturalist philosophies.

Robert Mendelsohn, M.D., (pp. 141-142) writes:

> There's no way anybody can justify the billions of dollars we spend every year on "health care." We're not getting healthier as the bill gets higher, we're getting sicker. Whether or not we have national health insurance is, at best, irrelevant and, at worst, one of the most dangerous decisions facing us in the years ahead. Because even if all doctors' services were free, disease and disability would not decrease.
>
> …Modern Medicine has succeeded in teaching us to equate *medical care* with *health*. It is that equation which has the potential to destroy our bodies, our families, our communities and our world.

MANUFACTURING MISCONCEPTIONS

With enough financial backing to create convincing advertising that appeals to the emotions of mass audiences, combined with strategic, frequent and repetitious commercial, infomercial and "news feature" airplay, special interest groups (such as the beef, dairy or drug industries) have been able to promote and proffer their products and services while fashioning a new reality in the Western world—the reality that certain *nonfoods* are nutritious, that we should live for today without regard for future illnesses, that we should rely on the quick fix concept of healthcare, and that nutrition runs secondary to taste in eating decisions. We are an "advanced" culture with NO means of prevention built into our formal education or healthcare system. The only institutions pushing for prevention are insurance companies, not because they want to see a healthy America and save us from the ravages of heart disease and cancer, but because illness is bad for their business. They want to figure out a way around having to give people their money back to pay for their medical bills.

PRACTICE PREVENTION & RESEARCH

The antidote to being the effect of big business is to practice prevention through good nutrition, supporting organic farmers, understanding your own body, and doing your own research. Find out the truth about health and disease, whether from a modern medical or natural healthcare perspective. The more aware you make yourself, the better decisions you will make.

EATING FOODS FOR ALL THE WRONG REASONS

According to *Whole Foods* magazine for the health food industry (1995, 20), even health food consumers make food choices primarily to satisfy their tastebuds, not their health. "Consumer research conducted for the Kushi Macrobiotics Corp. revealed that purchasers of popular branded health foods rate taste above health factors as their major reason for buying those products. According to the research, conducted by Evaluative Criteria, Inc., Stamford, good flavor and natural taste score higher as purchase motivators than low fat and cholesterol or other nutritional factors."

Use of the mass media by corporate entities has become an art form for dissemination of propaganda. Through the media—primarily television— seeds are planted for mass dependency on certain products and services with disregard for our state of health. These corporations perform a disservice to our culture, our country and society at large, and they are adept at keeping people from realizing the importance, if not the connection, between cause and effect relating to dietary intake and disease. When you see an advertisement, you may want to remind yourself that only a few short years ago ads proudly taught us that Camel cigarettes were the brand most doctors preferred to smoke. (Of course, advertisers are still using this tactic because it seems to work. Many commercials end with the words, "doctor recommended," or "the aspirin most doctors recommend," or "ask your doctor." Our medical doctors are strategically placed in the awkward position of indirectly endorsing products, from drugs to pillows and hemorrhoid creams to toothpaste).

To preserve your own state of health, remember that, to date, there is no replacement for the inherent balance and nutrition provided by nature. When man claims to improve upon nature, then common sense should shout to us from the rooftops to beware. Anything that is not natural (found in nature) poses a potential threat to life, human health and vitality.

TOXIC WASTES, FLUORIDE
& ENVIRONMENTAL THREATS TO HEALTH

The degree to which the inhabitants of this modern world are exposed to and affected by environmental and food-borne toxins is poorly understood and rarely recognized. Chemicals are ubiquitous in our lives—chemicals that destroy human, animal and plant health and continue to erode and unbalance our natural world and ecology. Large corporations dump their hazardous wastes into our waters, land and into the air while continuing to lie to the public about these practices and their dangers. As a result, we are battling with cancer and other diseases that overtake our immune systems. With strong, divisive public relations campaigns and media control, the general public is kept in the dark about poisons affecting our health and planet. Even President George W. Bush has played a role in purveying blatantly untrue and harmful messages to the American public when, during his campaign for presidency, he claimed that there is still "not enough evidence" to show the reality of global warming. This statement was made in defiance of the world's leading scientists, including those studying pictures taken from outer space showing the effects of global warming. His reason for making such an untruthful claim?—to protect his interests in oil drilling, natural gas and other profitable activities known to contribute to the problem of global warming and environmental destruction. Who will win out in the final battle? George Bush or Mother Nature?

FLUORIDE DANGER

America's top scientific researchers are coming forward to tell us that the fluoridation of our water was a big mistake, and that fluoride is a poisonous, industrial waste product that has NEVER been shown to reduce cavities or offer any health benefit. This is a very strong statement, and seems to go against the grain of what most Americans have been trained to think was the truth about fluoride, fluoride treatments at the dentist, fluoridated toothpaste, fluoride in foods, fluoride in carbonated soft drinks (*Journal of the American Dental Association*, November 1999) and fruit drinks, and fluoride in America's drinking water. Dentists have become pawns in this game of money and deceit, as they continue to promote the use of fluoride in their practices.

How did fluoride make its way into our hearts, minds and bodies? Following the Depression (1930s) the dental profession called for a solution to the great number of cavities rampant in America. Preliminary (but very faulty and inconclusive) studies pointed to the **theoretical possibility** of fluoride's role in decay prevention. Recently, Albert Burgstahler, Ph.D. (Organic Chemistry, Harvard University) gave a revealing interview in the publication *Acres, USA* (March, 2000) to confirm the slanted, faulty and unsubstantial claims that first led to the mass fluoridation of America's water supplies back in the 1940s. To the detriment of America's health, industries have been allowed by certain U.S. Government agencies (including the Public Health Service) to infuse our water supplies with the poisonous chemical known as fluoride.

Scientific tests repeatedly confirm that cities with high amounts of fluoride in their drinking water show no reduction of cavities among the residents. In fact, the opposite is true—decreased rates of cavities are found in non-fluoridated areas.

One-time strong advocate of fluoride use, Dr. Hardy Limbeback, University of Toronto, has had a change of mind and now concludes that "children under age three should not be using fluoridated water, beverages, baby formulas or any fluoride in any form. Because it's causing so much dental fluorosis in the tooth-forming stages," (*Acres, USA*, March 2000) as well as other systemic dangers for both children and adults of all ages.

ARE WE AN UNSUSPECTING OUTLET FOR INDUSTRIAL WASTE?

Dr. Burgstahler and Dr. Limeback suggest that the phosphate fertilizer industries use the public water systems as **an outlet for the waste byproducts of their industries.** When these industries make phosphate fertilizer, they start with rock phosphate (an apatite material) then treat it with concentrated sulfphuric acid to turn it into hydrogen phosphate. "But there is about two percent calcium fluoride in the apatite, and when you treat the apatite with sulphuric acid or even with phosphoric acid to make a superphosphate, hydrogen fluoride is eliminated, and that gas is too toxic to let go into the atmosphere, so it's put into holding ponds with silica, sand, and that converts it into fluorosilicic acid, which may be neutralized to get sodium fluorosilicate; and those are the two main chemicals sold for water fluoridation. Sodium fluorosilicate is a solid, powdery, poisonous material, and the hydrofuorosilicic acid is sold in rubber-lined tank cars at concentrations of around 26 percent and metered into water systems to get 1ppm fluoride"—**10 times the dosage originally approved for safety** by the American Waterworks Association in 1938.

Much research into fluoride should be garnered prior to believing this substance to be safe or even beneficial. The reader is urged to go online to fluoride.com for more information. Among some of the information found on this website:

- "fluoride may be linked to cancer."—*Newsweek,* Feb. 1990
- The American Medical Association states that it is "not prepared to state that fluoride is safe."—*AMA Letter*
- "fluoride damages bones at levels added to public drinking water."—*American Journal of Epidemiology*

- Since 1990, five major epidemiological studies show a high rate of hip fractures in fluoridated regions."—*Australian & New Zealand Journal of Public Health*
- "Hip fractures increased in areas with fluoridated water."—*Journal of American Medical Association*
- "Public health administrators should be aware of the total fluoride exposure before introducing any additional fluoride."—"Fluorides and Oral Health," Geneva, 1994)
- Dartmouth College conclusions find that "fluoridation is associated with an increase of lead levels in children"—280,000 children in this study.
- "Dentists cannot provide a medical opinion regarding the safety of ingested fluoride."—California Board of Dental Examiners
- **"Fluorides are general protoplasmic poisons**, probably because of their capacity to modify the metabolism of cells by changing the permeability of the cell membrane and by inhibiting certain enzyme systems."—*Journal of the American Medical Association*, Sept 18, 1943
- *"Segments of the population are unusually susceptible to the toxic effects of fluoride.* They include 'postmenopausal women and elderly men, pregnant woman and their fetuses, people with deficiencies of calcium, magnesium and/or vitamin C, and people with cardiovascular and kidney problems.' *United States Public Health Service Report* (ATSDR TP-91/17, pg. 112, Sec.2.7, April 1993)

WHAT CAN YOU DO ABOUT FLUORIDE?

Medical doctors, dentists in the know, scientific researchers and natural healthcare doctors urge everyone to learn as much as they can about fluoride & side effects, for health's sake. Discontinue using fluoride in toothpastes, drinking water, foods and drinks, and install a water filter at home and in the office. Moreover, many citizens have successfully lobbied and protested to have their cities ban fluoride in their water systems. Speaking out against fluoride, chlorination and other chemicals in your city's water supplies can garner positive outcomes.

TOXIC EFFECT OF SYNTHETIC FERTILIZERS

Following is a reprint of an article that ran in the *HealthxFiles Newsletter*, May 1998 (written by researchers at the Environmental Working Group) regarding the toxic effect of fertilizers upon our food supplies and farms. Exposure to environmental toxins is an ongoing concern in the face of corporate cover-ups of toxic waste dumping, chemical spills, the production and disposal of dangerous chemicals, the use of chemicals in foods and farming and the threat of a frightening array of chemicals impacting human health. Doctors specializing in environmental medicine are finding that many of the illnesses being blamed on viruses and bacteria are actually caused by exposure to toxic substances in the environment.

> **Toxic Wastes 'Recycled' as Fertilizer Threaten U.S. Farms and Food Supply Dioxin, Lead, Mercury Spread on Crops As States Scramble to Protect Public Health**
>
> [Washington, D.C.]—Under the guise of 'recycling,' millions of pounds of toxic waste are shipped each year from polluting industries to fertilizer manufacturers and farmers, who used toxic waste laden with dioxin, lead, mercury and other hazardous chemicals as raw material for fertilizers applied to U.S. farmland.
>
> According to an analysis of federal and state data released...by the Environmental Working Group (EWG), between 1990 and 1995 more than 450 fertilizer companies or farms in 38 states received shipments of toxic waste totaling more than 270 million pounds.
>
> EWG's report, Factory Farming: Toxic Waste and Fertilizers in the United States, lists, for each state, the polluting industries that shipped the most such waste and

the fertilizer companies that received the most. Companies in California received the most waste, followed by Nebraska, New Jersey, Washington, and Georgia.

"Not only does the EPA allow these chemicals to be used in the fertilizers that go on our crops, in most states farmers and consumers don't even have the right to know what's being used," said study author, Richard Wiles.

Because of loopholes in the federal toxics laws—most notably, the Toxics Release Inventory (TRI)—EWG found that it is impossible to account for all uses of the toxic waste shipped to fertilizer companies. "This is a regulatory system designed by Mr. Magoo," said Ken Cook, president of the Washington D.C.-based Environmental Working Group. Some facilities that received the waste only make fertilizer, but others produce a variety of inorganic chemicals.

However, in a series of investigative articles, *The Seattle Times* has documented the nationwide use of cadmium, lead, arsenic, dioxins, radionucleotides and other hazardous waste in fertilizer. Tests by the state of Washington found that some fertilizers contained very high levels of dioxin—100 times higher…than the level allowed for treated Superfund sites in the state.

In response to the *Seattle Times* investigation, states are scrambling to plug regulatory loopholes. Washington, California, Idaho, New Jersey, North Dakota, Maryland, Oklahoma, Oregon and Texas have laws or regulations in the works to limit toxic waste in fertilizer. Most of the proposals would still not provide consumers with as much information or put the burden on fertilizer companies to prove that their products are safe.

"Anyone who uses fertilizer has the right to know what is in it, and whether it was made from toxic waste," added Ken Cook, "But beyond this basic public right to know, state and federal health officials must protect farms, farm families and our food supply from toxic chemical contamination."

OTHER POISONOUS SUBSTANCES IN OUR LIVES & WHAT YOU CAN DO ABOUT THEM

The easiest way to avoid poisons in our foods is not to eat poisonous foods. For you and your family, purchase and eat only organically grown produce and meats. Organic foods are not drenched with synthetic fertilizers and chemical pesticides and infused with artificial ingredients such as refined sugars, food colorings, dyes, emulsifiers and other nonfood constituents. When eating at restaurants, demand organic foods. With enough demand, restaurateurs will consider such menu additions. For many years, the health food industry has been slandered, referring to natural foods as boring, unappetizing, "rabbit food," bland and unexciting. **This is a lie.** For every tasty poisoned food is a healthy, organic alternative without the chemicals. The choice is yours. (Refer to the Food Replacement List under the chapter "What's Left to Eat").

Other poisonous substances that lead to human disease that may be ingested by you and your family include:
- bug sprays/pesticides
- lawn fertilizers and pesticides
- paint, varnish, paint remover, gasoline fumes
- hair sprays
- personal toiletries such as perfumes, soaps, lotions and hair dyes
- plastic gasses
- barbecue cooking
- construction glues and degassing materials

- microwaves, aluminum cookware
- automobile and lawnmower pollution
- dishwasher soaps and detergents
- nuclear waste, plutonium waste in water and air
- industry waste in water, air and land

There are many more to add to this list, but this should get you thinking. Environmentalism is not for crackpots and "tree huggers," it has grown to become **the only sane force to oppose the giant corporations and utilities that affect us all with their arrogance, waste, perpetuation of lies and disregard for our health and habitat.**

EXCITOTOXINS IN FOODS?

Excitotoxins are flavor- and texture-enhancing chemicals added to a host of commercial, processed foods, the most infamous of which is MSG (monosodium glutamate) known for causing headaches to seizures, and most notably connected with Chinese restaurant foods. *Acres, USA* (February 2001) reported about the dangers of excitotoxins in foods in which Russell L. Blaylock, M.D., author of *Excitotoxins—the Taste that Kills*, explains how nerve cells in the brain are destroyed by synthetic glutamate-containing substances and shows how exposure to aluminum, and conditions of low blood sugar and deficiencies in magnesium and antioxidants, make people more vulnerable to the effects of MSG and related substances. Dr. Blaylock writes:

> 'What if someone were to tell you that a chemical added to food could cause brain damage in your children, and that this chemical could effect how your children's nervous systems formed during development so that in later years they might have learning or emotional difficulties? What if there was scientific evidence that these chemicals could damage a critical part of the brain known to control

hormones so that later in life your child might have endocrine problems? How would you fee?"

You would feel alarmed, deceived and angry.

Dr. Blaylock's critique of excitotoxins—MSG, hydrolyzed vegetable protein and aspartame—has raised some important consideration against the "continued adulteration of our food with these taste-enhancing substances":

> Babies and growing children are especially vulnerable to damage from synthetic glutamate containing substances, because their blood-brain barrier is not fully developed. MSG and the other excitotoxins can cause irreparable damage to the hypothalamus and glutamate-dependent nerve cells in several areas of the brain, yet MSG and hydrolyzed protein are routinely added to baby foods and other food items aimed at young children!
>
> Diets high in excitotoxins can cause learning disabilities, nervous disorders, seizures and hormonal imbalances in children. They are equally toxic to the elderly as they have been implicated as a major cause of the degenerative nervous disorders now afflicting adults with greater and greater frequency—Parkinson's, Alzheimer's, Lou Gehrig's and brain cancer. At any age, MSG, hydrolyzed protein and aspartame may cause headaches, seizures and allergic reactions in those who are sensitive.
>
> The volume of medical literature implicating excitotoxins is impressive—yet the FDA still allows their use in food. Worse, much MSG is not labeled and therefore remains hidden. Only pure MSG must be labeled…Foods containing hidden MSG include sodium caseinate, calcium caseinate, yeast extract, textured protein, autolyzed yeast, hydrolyzed flour, malt extract, malt flavoring, bouillon, broth, stock, "flavoring," "natural flavoring," "seasoning,"

"spices," carrageenan, enzymes, soy protein concentrate, soy protein isolate and whey protein concentrate. Various types of hydrolyzed protein are actually the precursors for MSG and are possibly more toxic.

THE ONE AND ONLY ECOLOGY

Most of us think of issues about pollution and wildlife when we hear the word "ecology." Yet this word should remind us that there is only one real ecology which pertains not only to our world and the environment, but also to our own bodily systems. As human beings—life forms living on the planet Earth—we are akin to our environment. Therefore, to live in health and balance, we demand clean air, water and soil; and we must have a clean body as well, free of toxic substances, environmental waste and harmful chemicals. We are interdependent, related creatures who cannot thrive in health by ingesting synthetic substances and by having our atmosphere destroyed by abuse that comes from corporate waste, air pollution, littering, nuclear waste dumping or the careless use and disposal of plastics.

OPENING UP TO SOLUTIONS
& THE DESIRE TO TAKE ACTION

If a "food" manufacturer made poison taste good, would people eat it? This is a rhetorical question, but the answer is a definitive "yes!" Every second of the day, in our affluent, highly-educated country, professors of science, doctors, surgeons, attorneys, heads of state, dietitians, ministers, musicians, fitness instructors, journalists, entertainers, and janitors all sit down to enjoy a tasty meal containing a wide array of pesticides, synthetic fertilizers, fluoride, chlorine, refined wheat, altered fats, refined sugar, artificial dyes, emulsifiers, fake fats, preservatives, MSG, chemicals and other poisons which take their toll on human health! Many of these ingredients are suspected of causing cancer, and many are *proven* to cause cancer. Still others may cause cancers when they interact with certain other chemicals found in processed food, conventionally grown fruits and vegetables, and the environment. These unnatural chemicals cause, or contribute to, all sorts of health problems, including headaches, nausea, skin eruptions, hormonal imbalances, PMS, heart disease, respiratory illnesses, tooth and gum disease, kidney and liver disease, etc. The fact that we are all exposed to poisons in our food and environment every day boggles the mind beyond mere words. This is a problem that did not exist a mere 200 years ago; it is a by-product of so-called "advancement" of our civilization and its technology.

THE DESIRE TO MAKE CHANGES

The difference between knowing you are being poisoned and actually doing something to stop the madness has to do with only one factor: **Desire to make a change for the better.** When we become aware of the existence of toxins in our lives and understand that we can take responsibility to ensure our health, it becomes extremely difficult to continue to accept and practice that which we know is wrong or unhealthful. Our eating decisions then may be no longer based on ignorance, taste and convenience, but rather on wisdom. This higher state of consciousness—or more enlightened way of looking at things—affords us the realization of how we need to make important choices in life, making it increasingly difficult to overlook the dangers of poisoned foods and continue to include them in our diet. With a higher state of consciousness, you free yourself to see past the illusion of advertising claims, brightly colored packaging and twisted marketing claims. The goal is to readily recognize the difference between a chemical and a food, and know that the chemical fails to meet the nutritional requirements of (and have the potential of harming) the cells in our bodies.

If you *desire* to make a change for the better (for the "healthier"), looking at your diet in a more critical fashion, refined foods lose their appeal and you begin to notice the taste, smell and feel of pesticide residues on non-organically grown produce. You come to realize that real apples picked from the tree are not excessively shiny, perfect-looking and evenly colored when they are grown naturally. With a greater appreciation for life and health, you'll notice that whole, natural foods taste better than processed non-foods; and the appeal of real food is that it is not masked by refined sugars, ketchup, excess salt or unnecessary. A higher state of awareness means breaking the chain of eating the same old foods you've always eaten out of habit, tradition and convenience despite their potential for harm. Let's face it: even if Mom's intentions were borne of love and devotion, she may have been unknowingly destroying our health. And it's a fact that most people continue to eat the same basic types of foods that they were raised on by their well-meaning mothers.

INCREASING YOUR AWARENESS

There's more to good health than just what meets the five senses. By developing our sense of awareness, corporations and special interest groups (with their self-serving agendas) lose their control over us. We begin to see the dangers of pesticides, toxic waste, radioactive materials, fluoride, nuclear energy, automobile and lawnmower exhaust, oil spills, inefficient electricity, chemical-laden foods, synthetically "vitamin" enriched foods, and harmful drugs. And we begin to detect the hidden messages and motives behind advertisements, news stories and marketing messages. Then we can regard our decisions based on whether we are contributing to the problem or proclaiming our harmony with nature and that which nurtures us.

Ironically, as one of the most "advanced" societies on earth, we constantly forfeit our sense of self-responsibility to mega-interest groups whose only goal is profit. While there is nothing wrong with capitalism and profit-making, there IS something wrong when corporations, institutions, and organizations capitalize on our hectic schedules, lack of understanding, fast-paced and segmented lifestyles and ignorance of human health to sell us health-destroying products. Making money at our expense is NOT okay. Making huge profits at the expense of our children's health is unconscionable. Metaphorically speaking, it's not that the sale of "snake oil" to the ignorant masses has disappeared from the scene—it has just become much more sophisticated; the flashy flim-flam man has been replaced with the flashy television commercial and so-called "news" exposé.

We need to take an objective look at ourselves and act in appreciation of the phenomenon of cause-and-effect. The emphasis in healing should not focus on "What will my doctor do for me?" but rather, "What can I do for myself with the help of a good doctor?"

Dr. Bernard Jensen (1984: IV) writes:

The consciousness of man today is not a healthy one. He comes to the office with bad habits; he knows practically nothing about the care of his body. As long as things are white, sterilized, clean and made by a well-known company, most people think the product should be good for them. This is a mistaken idea. We must consider our bodies as loyal servants depending upon our decisions, and know that everything that goes into the mouth as an effect upon them. Also, the body is affected by what you hear and see, by your feelings—and it can all add up to our good or to our destruction. All of these things should be understood.

As a primer, every novice to natural healthcare should read Dr. Jensen's *Vibrant Health From Your Kitchen*.

LIVING IN A STATE OF BALANCE

Deepak Chopra, M.D. (1994: 45) tells us that the law of cause and effect, "says no debt in the universe ever goes unpaid. There is a perfect system in this universe, and everything is a constant 'to and fro' exchange of energy."

Without considering the cause of illness—or any problem we face—we never actually get to the bottom of it and find that it is bound to resurface in another way and at another time. Thus, the foundation is paved for failure to achieve lasting health as well as the destiny to repeat the patterns which originally led to the diseased state in the first place. We come to understand why the smoker who has a heart attack returns to his cigarette habit, the drug abuser or alcoholic rehabilitates only to fall out of grace with himself and society once again, overweight people lose weight and then default to their "old selves" a year later, etc. It takes more than just agreeing with the principles of natural healthcare to eradicate the ills in our lives and all around us; it takes a dedicated effort and desire to make changes.

TOOLS FOR BECOMING MORE AWARE

To make a lasting change in your health is to break the pattern of living *reactively*—by allowing things to happen *before* taking notice of the problem. Methods (tools) for accomplishing this include meditation and self study to become more aware and accepting of each "clue" life gives you to expand your understanding of its myriad systems. Actively practicing meditative types of exercises is supportive to anyone desiring to increase awareness, just as exercising the muscles is essential for anyone determined to compete in athletics. And the side effect of meditation is stress-relief. Conscious growth comes from desire to learn and putting that education into practice. There are countless books, essays, discourses, audiotapes and classes teaching people the "mechanics" of meditation, as well as how to live a healthier life, how to eat naturally, how to live without toxic chemicals and how to cope with stress. This is an ongoing process as you journey through life.

Find a method of learning that works comfortably for you, one which brings all of the scattered aspects of yourself into wholeness—the physical, emotional, mental and spiritual parts of your life. Expanding your awareness and living in harmony with nature allows you to integrate these aspects of yourself into one unified self. In so doing, it will become easier not to let your tastebuds make dietary choices for you, not to allow stress to influence you into attacking a half gallon of ice cream and refusing to let advertising commercials and corporate propaganda set misleading standards for "healthy" eating and lifestyle.

Dr. Bernard Jensen writes (1984; 33), "No part of the physical body or cell in the body can be divorced from the spirit, that life force that flows through us. The more highly evolved man becomes, the more he recognizes that changes in consciousness rid him of sickness and make him 'whole' once again."

HEALTH CONSCIOUSNESS

Of course it is a necessary first step to understand how and what to eat for the sake of good health, but the next step is to actually become health conscious (aware of your state of health and the desire to take responsibility for it). This involves incorporating your knowledge, senses, experience, instincts and intuition into your decision-making processes and applying them to work toward health and happiness. Health consciousness means creating and embracing healthful thoughts and attitudes which become a part of you instead of just facts and figures stored in your memory like an unopened guidebook to life, collecting dust on some seldom-visited library shelf. Health consciousness is practical and active, not static and theoretical. You need more than just information to become healthy; you need to actively pursue good health.

Cardiologist Dean Ornish, M.D. (Moyers, 1993: 95) writes,

> Providing people with health information is important, but it's not usually enough to motivate lasting changes in behavior unless we also deal with the more fundamental issues that motivate us. Working at that level brings us to the psycho-social and even spiritual dimensions…When people learn to experience inner peace—when we work on that level—then they are more likely to make and maintain lifestyle choices that are life-enhancing rather than self-destructive.

The dynamics of what motivates people to change their eating patterns is explored in Ornish's studies with cardiac patients. Ornish (Moyers, 1994; 97) says, "if you make comprehensive changes in diet and lifestyle…you begin to feel so much better so quickly that the choices become clear and you may say, 'Yeah, I really like eating meat all the time, but I like the way I feel now so much better, that the choice not to eat meat is worth it to me.'

Ornish continues:

One of the patients in our [cardiac/heart] study had severe chest pains whenever he tried to work, make love with his wife, or exercise. Now he can do all of these without pain. He said, 'I like eating meat—but not that much.'

Most health practitioners try to motivate people to change out of fear—you're going to be dead if you don't change; you're going to get a heart attack; you're a time bomb—all these terrible images. That doesn't work very well...Although we know at some level that we may get sick and die, it is too terrifying to think about, and so we tend to deny it. For the first one or two weeks after someone's had a heart attack, you have their full attention. Then the denial begins, and you lose it... Efforts to motivate people to change out of fear don't work very long.

DON'T GIVE UP ON YOURSELF
—MINOR SETBACKS

In the field of natural healthcare, we can't afford to get lost in idealism or create unrealistic expectations or goals. We are all human, subject to emotional ups and downs, setbacks, laziness, fear, confusion, stress and forgetfulness. There are times when we just can't resist eating a half dozen cookies, even if it's just to remind us that it gives us a splitting headache the next morning. Any person on the journey to better health through nutrition comes to appreciate that there may be occasional lapses into eating inharmonious foods. However, with a lifestyle dedicated to a healthier purpose, there is less likelihood that such lapses will be permanent and lead to a total reversion to poor lifestyle habits. We can't afford to be so hard on ourselves that we end up like the dieter who surrenders in disgust at his own fallibility and regains 50 pounds in a fit of hopeless depression. This is a slow, steady, deliberate growth process that requires patience with yourself. It is a journey fueled NOT by discipline, but by *motivation*. Discipline uses force to achieve your goals; motivation comes from love, desire and inspiration. Deepak Chopra, M.D. tells us (1995; 89), "When you *force* solutions on problems, you only create new problems."

SELF RESPONSIBILITY

Taking responsibility for our actions is a foreign concept to most of us in this modern society, especially pertaining to our eating habits and physical health. Our state of health is surrendered to doctors, institutions, restaurants and government agencies entrusted to act in our best interest. Dr. Herbert L. Ley, Jr., former FDA (Food & Drug Administration) commissioner (Bliss, 137) said, "The thing that bugs me is that the people think the FDA is protecting them—it isn't. What the FDA is doing and what the public thinks it is doing are as different as night and day." The solution: Trust yourself, trust your own research, trust nature.

Forfeiting personal responsibility as a cultural way of life has given rise to our pollution, crime, legal system, politics, environmental and moral degradation, modern farming methods, strip mining, nuclear waste creation and disposal, chemical dumping, misleading advertising, nutritional decline, an out-of-control welfare system, a national deficit, a failing educational system, unregulated mass communications and our personal and national ill state of health. Quite ironically, we have learned to surrender the most important decisions affecting our very vitality to outside forces. In so doing, we have removed ourselves so far from the *effect* of our actions that we are missing the lessons of life; we cannot see the delicate balance linking cause with effect, action with reaction, exposure to toxins with illness, and diet with disease.

As spiritual, thinking beings, we find health and happiness in freedom. By surrendering our freedom to outside influences, we become unhappy and unhealthy. We cannot afford the consequences of surrendering our food choices to self-centered corporations, hectic schedules that lead us to dine out four to five times a week at unhealthy restaurants, or to "respectable" private institutions and government agencies which betray our trust in favor of their profit margins.

AN EXACTING SYSTEM

If you are interested in changing your eating and lifestyle habits for a healthier you, then recognize that what you do today affects your life tomorrow, whether your actions pertain to the way you speak to others or what you eat for breakfast. To work within this system, seek to balance yourself by assuming conscious actions, thoughts and intentions. See yourself as part of the flow of the lifestream, instead of a helpless victim of its awesome current, or worse, a perpetrator of illness. To do this, you must act with total responsibility and understand that you have control over your choices to create negative actions, positive actions and inactions. If you act without thinking, life doesn't let you off the hook so easily.

Chopra (1995; 40) explains

> You and I are essentially infinite choice-makers. In every moment of our existence, we are in that field of all possibilities where we have access to an infinity of choices. Some of these choices are made consciously, while others are made unconsciously. But the best way to understand and maximize the use of karmic law [principle of cause and effect] is to become consciously aware of the choices we make in every moment....If you step back for a moment and witness the choices you are making...then in just this act of witnessing, you take the whole process from the unconscious realm into the conscious realm. This procedure of conscious choice-making and witnessing is very empowering.

Dr. Bernard Jensen (*Vibrant Health From Your Kitchen*) writes:

> "I believe man wants to do what is right and will, if shown that doing the right thing will result in a better life."

CONCLUSIONS

Natural Healthcare is a blossoming field of rediscovery.

After millions of years of "practicing" natural healthcare, mankind took a brief detour onto the road of Modern Medicine and its system of drugs, chemicals, injections, surgeries, hospitals and monopolization of healthcare to the detriment of freedom, democracy, personal rights and recovery and prevention. To further complicate matters, within the past couple of generations we have witnessed the mass destruction of our daily diets and health with the institution of food processing and ubiquitous use of chemicals that have replaced real, natural foods and natural BIOchemicals, respectively. Such so-called "advancements" in technology continue to destroy our personal health, environment and peace-of-mind. A return to Nature is the "natural" antithesis to the chronic illness we have experienced under artificial conditions.

At long last, over the past two decades we have seen a renewed commitment and appreciation for natural healing, natural treatments, natural healthcare settings and the ingestion of natural substances such as herbs, whole food supplements and organic foods. We have also—in spite of the efforts of the modern medical giant to keep us dependent on its trinity of drugs, medical doctors and hospitals—taken our health into our own hands, realizing that good health is not the absence of disease, but rather a natural state of being; and that doctors should be our servants, not the other way around. Even medical doctors have moved beyond the "party line" and have joined in this movement toward natural solutions to chronic illness.

Natural healthcare is an approach that, unlike the modern medical model, incorporates not just treatments for disease, but more importantly, wisdom of prevention, lifestyle habits, organic farming, emotional and mental balance, dietary choices, environmental issues and self responsibility. There is an emerging recognition, by those whose better sense of judgment is not dominated by their egos or pocketbooks, of the fact that there is not one sole mode of healing or therapy befitting any one of us. And there is once again a revival in the wisdom of ancient forms of treatment, including Traditional Chinese Medicine, massage, nutrition, exercise, meditation, and so on. Modern civilization has given the modern medical system a try and it has failed miserably to eradicate the plagues of our era (cancer, arthritis, heart disease, etc.), prevent illness and impress upon us the importance of living in harmony with our environment. Now we are once again giving Nature a try because we are waking up to the fact that her awesome complexity for nurturing life can never be duplicated by science.

ABOUT THE AUTHOR

Vic Shayne, Ph.D., is a doctors' consultant, food science researcher, lecturer, and whole food supplement formulator. Dr. Shayne has been a writer for the past 22 years on topics ranging from natural healthcare to disease etiology. He is a nutritionist, herbologist, Chinese Lymphatic Massage therapist and a practitioner of Chinese Qigong. He is the past director of the Holistic Health & Counseling Center in Carefree, Arizona and is a professor of clinical nutrition at the University of Natural Medicine, New Mexico. Dr. Shayne is also the editor of *HealthXFiles Newsletter*, *Clinical Nutritionist Newsletter* and *ROOTS Newsletter for Natural Healthcare Practitioners*, as well as the author of *Whole Food Nutrition: The Missing Link in Vitamin Therapy*. Vic Shayne bases his healthcare philosophy on naturalist principles in harmony with the body's biochemistry and physiology, and the environment; and decision-making processes predicated on awareness.

PRODUCT RESOURCE GUIDE

Supplements
NATURE'S WELLNESS CENTER
www.natureswellness.com
Dr. Russell W. Shurtleff, DC, FIACA
Scottsdale, Arizona
1-800-294-6686

Nature's Wellness Center is an excellent source for whole food complex supplements, essential fatty acids, wheat germ oil (for natural vitamin E), detoxification products and more. Nature's Wellness also offers telephone consultations for patients needing nutritional support and individually-designed healthcare programs. Dr. Shurtleff offers a HealthScan patient survey that can be filled out at home and mailed or faxed in. Also available: informative materials on natural healthcare issues and health-promoting products including air and water filters. Dr. Shurtleff works with patients' medical doctors, chiropractors, nutritionists and other professionals to evaluate blood tests, urine tests, hair mineral analyses, etc.

NUTRIPLEX FORMULAS, INC.
(www.nutriplexformulas.com)
1-888-595-4752 doctor's orders only

NutriPlex Formulas, Inc. formulates whole food complexes sold only through doctors practicing natural healthcare and clinical nutrition worldwide. Products contain vitamins and minerals still intact within their original, natural and undisturbed food complex along with enzymes, coenzymes, essential fatty acids, phytonutrients, trace minerals, etc. If you are interested in NutriPlex's products, contact your doctor for information. Available through NutriPlex Formulas, Inc. is ROOTS newsletter for professional healthcare practitioners needing biochemical facts to support clinical nutrition practices.

Newsletters
CREATIVE BUREAU, INC.
ROOTS Newsletter
(Mail Order Only)
P.O. Box 17482, Boulder, CO 80308

Publishes newsletters healthcare practitioners non-professionals offering biochemical facts about healthcare and nutrition, and mind-body healthcare. Articles are written by professionals with clinical experience in biochemistry, clinical nutrition, psychology, hypnotherapy, chiropractic, and transpersonal counseling. Articles keep readers abreast of information on supplements, specific illnesses and nutrients which support the body, the role of the mind in the healing process, immunity, toxicity in the environment and food supplies, etc. Creative Bureau publications offer information not influenced by advertisers, fads or marketing claims.

Courses
UNIVERSITY OF NATURAL MEDICINE
Santa Fe, New Mexico
Dr. Mark D. Smith (ND)
1-800-893-3367
www.unaturalmed.edu
Offers courses on natural healthcare, nutrition, naturopathic and alternative health. Regionally accredited courses available through the mail with experienced professors.

Herbs
STARWEST BOTANNICALS, INC.
11253 Trade Center Drive
Rancho Cordova, CA 95742
1-800/800-4372
Organically grown herbs and herbal formulations.

NATURE'S WELLNESS CENTER
www.natureswellness.com
Dr. Russell W. Shurtleff, DC, FIACA
Scottsdale, Arizona
1-800-294-6686

Grow Your Own Herbs
AMERICAN GINSENG GARDEN
Box 400 Mountain Meadow Lane
Flag Pond, TN 37657

FRONTIER HERBS
3021 78th Street
P.O. Box 299
Norway, IA 52318

NORTHWOODS RETAIL NURSERY
27635 S. Oglesby Road
Canby, OR 97013

PACIFIC BOTANNICALS
4350 Fish Hatchery Road
Grants Pass, OR 97527

Health Food Stores
WILD OATS
ALFALFA'S
Boulder, Colorado headquarters
Nationwide

Wild Oats is a national healthfood chain committed not only to providing natural, organic foods, but also environmental and consumer issues such as organic farming. Thus far, the company's management has been responsive to customer input and demand for quality healthcare products and foods.

Health Food Mail Order
WALNUT ACRES
1-800-433-3998
Penns Creek, Pennsylvania 17862-0800

Walnut Acres is a provider of organically grown produce from their farms in Pennsylvania. Their products are available by mail nationwide. Also included in the Walnut Acres catalog are organic sauces, herbs & spices, syrup, honey, dried fruit, household products, bath & beauty aids and more.

Nutrition for Pets
SHERRY PIERNICK, 1-719-487-0525
DR. HENRY PASTERNAK (DVM): 310-454-2917
Whole food concentrate supplementation for dogs, cats and other carnivorous animals made without preservatives, isolated vitamins or minerals. All natural, concentrated real foods in a powder form, endorsed by holistic veterinarian, Henry Pasternak, DMV, Pacific Pallisades, California.

READING RESOURCE GUIDE

The following books, magazines and tapes contain valuable information worthy of consideration for those seeking a healthier lifestyle. The reader is advised to keep an open mind to discern for him/herself the value of these publications. Those materials listed with an asterisk (*) are highly recommended. All resources noted are worthy of consideration due to their earnest commitment to natural healthcare or environmental concerns. However, this author does not recommend the use of fractionated/isolated or synthetic vitamin and mineral supplements that may be mentioned in any of the recommended books. Whole food supplements are the better alternative.

ALTERNATIVE MEDICINE THE DEFINITIVE GUIDE
Future Medicine Publishing
10124 18th Street, Court E
Puyallup, WA 98317
Encyclopedia of Alternative Therapies

* THE DETOX DIET
Elson Haas, M.D.
Celestial Arts
Berkeley, CA, 1996

*DIET FOR A NEW WORLD
John Robbins
Avon Books
New York, 1992

DR. WRIGHT'S GUIDE TO HEALING WITH NUTRITION
Jonathan V. Wright, M.D.
Keats Publishing, Inc.
New Canaan, CT 1990

*THE COMPLETE BOOK OF JUICING
Michael T. Murray, N.D.
Prima Health,
Roseville, CA 1998

*E THE ENVIRONMENTAL MAGAZINE
P.O. Box 2947
Marion, OH 43306
813-734-1242

EAT MORE, WEIGH LESS
Dean Ornish, M.D.
Harper Perennial
New York, 1994

THE ENCYCLOPEDIA OF NUTRITION & GOOD HEALTH
Robert A. Ronzio, Ph.D., CNS, FAIC
Facts on File, Inc.
New York, 1997

*EMPTY HARVEST
Dr. Bernard Jensen
Bernard Jensen Publisher
Escondido, CA 1993

*FOODS THAT HEAL
Bernard Jensen, D.C., Ph.D.
Avery Publishing
Garden City Park, NY 1993

HEINERMAN'S ENCYCLOPEDIA OF FRUITS, VEGETABLES & HERBS
John Heinerman
Parker Publishing Co.
West Nyack, NY 1988

NATIONAL GREEN PAGES
Directory of Environmental & Socially Responsible Companies
Annual: Washington, DC 202/872-5307

*NATURE HAS A REMEDY
Bernard Jensen, D.C., Ph.D.
Bernard Jensen International
Escondido, CA 1981

REVERSING HEART DISEASE
Dean Ornish, M.D.
Ballantine Books
New York, 1990

I have X (handwritten)

*ROOTS NEWSLETTER
A concise publication for professionals and nonprofessionals featuring bio-chemical facts on nutrition and health, and mind-body healthcare articles: $25 per year, bi-monthly, 8 pages.
Creative Bureau, Inc., P.O. Box 17231, Boulder, Colorado 80308

*"SABOTAGING THE HEALTH OF AMERICA"
Audiotape
Send $3 to
Dr. Vic Shayne
Creative Bureau, Inc.
P.O. Box 17482, Boulder, CO 80308
This tape explains the use of whole food complex supplements in the author's personal experience both as a patient and as a practitioner.

*SAFE SHOPPERS BIBLE
David Steinman
MacMillian USA
New York 1995

SECOND OPINION NEWSLETTER
William Campbell Douglass, M.D.
Monthly newsletter
Atlanta, GA: 800/728-2288

* 20 YEARS OF CENSORED NEWS
A concise resource of important news information that the general public rarely hears about, yet adversely affects our quality of life and threatens individual freedoms.
Carl Jensen, Ph.D.
Seven Stories Press, New York, 1997

*UNDERSTANDING FATS & OILS:
YOUR GUIDE TO HEALING WITH ESSENTIAL FATTY ACIDS
Michael T. Murray, N.D. & Jade Beutler, RRT, RCP
Progressive Health Publishing
Encinitas, CA 1996

* WHOLE FOOD NUTRITION: The Missing Link in Vitamin Therapy
Vic Shayne, Ph.D.
This book contains scientific research and clinical experience proving the viability of whole food complexes in food and supplement form versus so-called vitamins. Well documented research explaining how whole food concentrate supplements are present within a "complex" which supplies not only vitamins, but also enzymes, amino acids, protein, minerals, trace minerals, coenzymes and other synergistic food factors in their original, balanced ratios.
Available through Barnes & Noble stores, www.bn.com, or your local book retailer.
ISBN # 595144764
iUniverse Publishing, 2000

BIBLIOGRAPHY

Acres, USA, Austin, TX, issues: 2000-2001

Acres, USA, Russell L. Blaylock, M.D., Austin, TX, February 2001

Ballantine, M.D., Rudolph, *Diet & Nutrition, A Holistic Approach,* 1978. Himalayan International Institute, Homesdale, PA

Belkin, Lisa, "Primetime Pushers," *Mother Jones,* March/April 2001

Berkow, M.D., Robert (Ed.), *The Merck Manual of Diagnosis & Therapy,* 1992, Merck Research Laboratories, Rahway, NJ

Bliss, Shepard, *The New Holistic Handbook* 1985, Stephen Greene Press, Lexington, MA

Bozich, Tim, *Basic Chemistry,* 1972, Prentice Hall, NJ

Burrows, Marion, "Additives In Advice On Food?", *The New York Times,* Nov. 15, 1995

Buist, Robert, Ph.D., *Food Chemical Sensitivity,* 1988, Avery Publishing, NY

Campt, Doug, "A Look at the Basics: Reducing Dietary Risk," *EPA Journal,* 1990, May/June

Chevallier, Andrew, *The Encyclopedia of Medicinal Plants,* 1996, DK Publishing, Inc., NY

Chopra, M.D., Deepak, *The 7 Spiritual Laws of Success,* 1994, Amber Allen Publishing, San Rafael, CA

Colbin, Annemarie, *Food & Healing,* Ballentine Books, NY, 1996

Collin, M.D., Jonathan, *Townsend Newsletter for Doctors,* 1995, Jonathan Collins, M.D., Publisher, Port Townsend, WA

Dadd, Debra Lynn, *Home Safe Home,* 1997, Penguin Putnam, NY

DeCava, MS, LNC, Judith A., "Digestive Physiology—A Review," Adjunctive Tips, 1988, Vol 4, No.31

DeCava, MS, LNC, Judith A., "Pesticides: What Goes Around Comes Around," *The Wellness Advocate*, 1994, Vol.1 No.2

Duke, Ph.D., James, *The Green Pharmacy*, Rodale Press, Pennsylvania, 1997

E Environmental Magazine (March/April 2001, pp. 12-13)

Erasmus, Udo, *Fats That Heal, Fats That Kill*, 1993, Alive Books, Vancouver, Canada

Finnegan, John, *The Facts About Fats*, Celestial Arts, Berkeley, CA 1993

Funk, Ph.D., Joel, "Naturopathic & Allopathic Healing, A Developmental Comparison," *Townsend Newsletter for Doctors & Patients*, October 1995, Jonathan Collin, M.D., Publisher, Port Townsend, WA

Giller, M.D., Robert M., *Natural Prescriptions*, 1994, Ballantine Books, NY

Gawain, Shakti, "Creative Visualization," Whatever Publishing, Oakland, CA 1978

Glazer, Sarah, "How America Eats," Editorial Research Reports, *Congressional Quarterly*, 1988, April, Vol. 1, No. 16

Goldberg, Burton, *Alternative Medicine: The Definitive Guide* 1994, Future Medicine Publishing, Inc., Duyallup, WA

Goldberg, Burton, *The Alternative Medicine Digest* 1994, Future Medicine Publishing, Inc., Duyallup, WA

Goldbeck, David, "How to Read a Food Label," *Mother Earth News*, 1989, March/April

Gottlieb, William, Ed., *Intensive Healing Diets*, 1988, Rodale Press, Emmaus, PA

Haas, M.D., Elson, *The Detox Diet*, Celestial Publishing, Berkeley, CA, 1996

Haas, M.D., Elson, *The False Fat Diet*, Ballantine Books, NY 2000

Haas, M.D., Elson, *Staying Healthy With Nutrition,* Celestial Publishing, Berkeley, CA, 1999

Health News & Review, 1995 Keats Publishing, New Canaan, CT

Health Foods Business. "Back Talk," 1995, May

Heinermann, John, *Heinermann's Encyclopedia of Fruits, Vegetables & Herbs*, 1988, Parker Publishing Co, West Nyak, NY

Holmes, Hannah, "Eating Low on the Food Chain," *Garbage*, 1992, January/February

Howell, Dr. Edward, *Enzyme Nutrition, The Food Enzyme Concept*, 1988, Avery Publishing Group, Inc.

Jensen, Ph.D., Carl, *20 Years of Censored News*, 1997, Seven Stories Press, New York

Jensen, D.C., Ph.D., Bernard, *Doctor-Patient Handbook*, 1976, Bernard Jensen Enterprises, Escondido, CA

Jensen, D.C., Ph.D., Bernard, *Empty Harvest*, 1994, Avery Publishing Group, Garden City, NY

Jensen, D.C., Ph.D., Bernard, Foods That Heal, 1993, Avery Publishing Group, Garden City, NY

Jensen, D.C., Ph.D., Bernard, *How to Enjoy Better Health With Natural Remedies*, 1980, Bernard Jensen Products, Escondido, CA

Jensen, D.C., Ph.D., Bernard, *The Joy of Living & How to Attain It*, 1970, Bernard Jensen Products, Solana Beach, CA

Jensen, D.C., Ph.D., Bernard, *Master Feeding Program*, 1988, Bernard Jensen Enterprises, Escondido, CA

Jensen, D.C., Ph.D., Bernard, *Nature Has a Remedy*, 1984, Dr. Bernard Jensen, Escondido, CA

Jensen, Ph.D., Bernard, *Nutrition Handbook*, 1993, Bernard Jensen, Ph.D., Escondido, CA

Jones, Heather, "Diet & Health: Ten Megatrends," *Nutrition Action Healthletter*, January/February Washington, DC, 2001

Kouchakoff, M.D., Paul, "The Influence of Food Cooking on the Blood Formula of Man," Institute of Clinical Chemistry, Lousanne, Switzerland, *Journal of the National Academy of Research Biochemists*, November/December, 1992

Lee, Ph.D., Lita, "Enzyme Nutrition Part I—Nutritional Myths," *Townsend Letter for Doctors*, 1992, April

Mason, M.S., Russ, "Questioning Conventional Oncology," *Alternative Complementary Therapies*, Vol. 7, No. 1, February 2001

McGuire, Meredith B., "The New Spirituality: Healing Rituals Hit the Suburbs," *Psychology Today*, 1989, January/February

Mendelsohn, M.D., Robert S., *Confessions of a Medical Heretic*, Contemporary Books, Chicago, 1979.

Moyers, Bill, *Healing & The Mind*, 1993, Doubleday, New York

Murray, Dr. Richard P., "Food Enzymes," *Applications in Human Nutrition*, Biomedical Health Foundation, Vol. 1, No. 1, Part A, 1990, Arnold, MO, Vol. 1, No. 1, Part B, Pace, Florida

Murray, Dr. Richard P., *Biomedical Nitty Gritty*, Biomedical Health Foundation, "Stress," July-August, 1986, Ocala, Florida, Biomedical Health Foundation

Murray, D.C., Richard P., "B Complex Deficit Syndrome," January-February 1984, "Natural vs. Synthetic,"

Murray, D.C., P.A., Richard P., January 1982, "Implanted Concepts," Murray, D.C., P.A., Richard P., August 1982

Murray, Dr. Richard P., *The Clinical Nutritionist Newsletter*, "Consistent Inconsistencies," 1985, National Academy of Research Biochemists, Vol. 6, No. 3, Biloxi, MS

NutriPlex Formulas, Inc. Website, 1998, www.nutriplexformulas.com

Ornish, M.D., Dean, *Eat More, Weigh Less*, 1994, Harper Perennial, New York

Ornish, M.D., Dean, *Reversing Heart Disease*, 1990, Ballentine Books, New York

Pauling, Linus, *Vitamin C, The Common Cold & The Flu*, 1981, Berkeley Books, New York

Peck, M.D., M. Scott, *The Road Less Traveled*, 1978, Simon & Shuster, New York

Petrovsky, Fred, "Setting the Record Straight on Vitamin Supplements, *Vim & Vigor*, 1992, Spring

The Record, Section A-31, December 3, 1992, Hackensack, NJ

Reid, Daniel, *The Complete Book of CHINESE Health & Healing*, 1994, Shambhala Publications, Boston

Reuben, M.D., David, *The Save Your Life Diet*, 1975, Random House, New York

Robbins, John, *Diet for a New World*, 1992, Avon Books, New York

Ronzio, Ph.D., CNS, FAIC, Robert A., *The Encyclopedia of Nutrition & Good Health*, 1997, Facts on File, NY

Shayne, Ph.D., Vic, *Whole Food Nutrition: The Missing Link in Vitamin Therapy*, 2000, iUniverse, New York

Shayne, Ph.D., Vic, *ROOTS Newsletter for Natural Healthcare Practitioners*, "Is High Potency 'Natural,' or Pharmacological?" Vol. 4, No. 4, 1998, Creative Bureau, Inc., Carefree, AZ

Santillo, N.D., Humbart, *Natural Healing With Herbs*, 1993, Hohm Press, Prescott, Arizona

Shelton, Herbert M., *Food Combining Made Easy*, 1992, Willow Publishing, San Antonio, TX

Stone, Eden, "Good-bye to Beef," *New Age Journal*, 1992, March/June

Thibodeau, Gary A., *Anthony's Textbook of Anatomy & Physiology*, 13th Edition, Times Mirror/Mosby College Publishing, St. Louis, MO

Winter, Ruth, *A Consumer's Dictionary of Food Additives*, 1994, Three Rivers Press, New York

Whitaker, M.D., Julian, *Health & Healing*, January 1995 Supplement, "The American Dietetic Association Must be Stopped in its Tracks," Phillips Publishing, Inc.

Whole Foods, "Newslinks," 1995, June

Wright, M.D., Jonathan V., *Dr. Wright's Guide to Healing with Nutrition*, 1984, Keats Publishing, New Canaan, CT

INDEX

Printed in the United States
40453LVS00004B/7